EVERY DAY
IS GAME DAY

EVERY DAY
IS GAME DAY

Train Like the Pros With a No-Holds-Barred
Exercise and Nutrition Plan for Peak Performance

MARK VERSTEGEN

AND PETE WILLIAMS

Authors of *Core Performance*

AVERY
a member of Penguin Group (USA)
New York

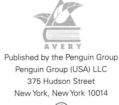

Published by the Penguin Group
Penguin Group (USA) LLC
375 Hudson Street
New York, New York 10014

USA • Canada • UK • Ireland • Australia
New Zealand • India • South Africa • China

penguin.com
A Penguin Random House Company

First trade paperback edition 2014
Copyright © 2014 by Athletes' Performance, Inc.
Exercise images courtesy of Dave Schifrin

Most Avery books are available at special quantity discounts for bulk purchase for sales promotions, premiums, fund-raising, and educational needs. Special books or book excerpts also can be created to fit specific needs. For details, write Special.Markets@us.penguingroup.com.

The Library of Congress has catalogued the hardcover edition as follows:

Verstegen, Mark, date.
Every day is game day : the proven system of elite performance to win all day, every day /
Mark Verstegen, Pete Williams.
p.   cm.
Includes bibliographical references and index.
ISBN 978-1-58333-516-1
1. Bodybuilding.   2. Exercise.   I. Williams, Pete, 1969–   II. Title.
GV546.5V48   2014   2013030287
613.7'13—dc23
ISBN 978-1-58333-553-6 (paperback)

Printed in the United States of America
1   3   5   7   9   10   8   6   4   2

BOOK DESIGN BY TANYA MAIBORODA

To the athletes, staff, peers, and predecessors
in the field, and the extended family of Athletes' Performance.
We are ONE team, united in the goal of supporting one another
to embrace and meet every challenge, succeed in every mission,
exceed every expectation, and relentlessly drive ourselves
and future generations to higher levels of success.
All day. Every day.

Contents

EVERY DAY
IS GAME DAY

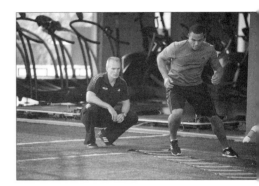

Introduction:
Your Performance Day

YOUR BEST ISN'T GOOD ENOUGH.

That sounds harsh, and indeed it is. But having worked with the best of the best over the last two decades, I've learned what it takes to be the best.

Anyone can hit excellence for a day, even a week or a month. That's easy. But a high performer is one who does it consistently for years over the course of a career.

You can be talented, work hard, and do all the right things, and it might not be enough. Not anymore. These days, performance is about results. It's not just showing up every day, working hard, and doing the right things. That's great. That's expected. Performance is about showing up every day and hitting the bull's-eye regardless of the situation.

That's performance.

Performance is about efficiency. If you've picked up this book, you're either a high performer looking to take things up a notch or someone aspiring to be a high performer. Regardless of who you are, you need to become more efficient in every aspect of your life in order to sustain that high performance and raise the bar every day.

That's why your best isn't good enough. I don't care who you are. My best is not good enough. It's not good enough for my family, my colleagues, or my country. It might have been sufficient yesterday or last year. But it won't be good enough for tomorrow or next year. Instead, what will make us high performers is how relentlessly we hone our lives every day to become smarter and more efficient.

24/7.

This book is not about a one-hour daily workout. That's the easy part, though you might disagree during the training portion of this program. The challenge is living a high-performance lifestyle the other twenty-three hours. Can you hit benchmarks over the course of your day, well beyond the gym? That's what it takes to be an elite performer.

Once you install the process you will learn and follow in this book, it becomes part of you, your new normal. High performers always are creating a new norm that was better than where they were a year ago or even last week.

That's why this is not a traditional training book. Yes, you will learn scientifically proven performance strategies to receive huge ROI—both a return on investment (of time) *and* a reduction of injury.

There's a lot to be said for investing an hour or so a day to obtain such a return on investment. Compound interest is a powerful thing. That's why we don't think of training as only what's accomplished in the gym. What about the other twenty-three hours of your day? What about all those little daily opportunities, some perhaps only a few minutes or even just seconds, to help you achieve your high-performance life?

Think of training not in physical terms, but rather as the *process* of what it takes to bring your A-game all day, every day, to hit your goals, whatever they might be. We're not here to excel in sports, though perhaps that's a goal for you, but rather to thrive in all aspects of our lives.

For the people we deal with at Athletes' Performance, a group that includes the world's most elite athletes and the world's most elite fighting forces, working hard and doing the right things often are not enough. This applies even when you're the most talented. We want you to "piss excellence" in everything you do.

What makes the difference is identifying the inefficiencies in your life and relentlessly honing them to become more efficient. We want to become more efficient in every aspect of our lives.

When we realize that Every Day Is Game Day and approach it accordingly, we win. When we're able to establish this integrated, efficient, twenty-four-hour lifestyle system for sustainable high performance, then we're well on our way to creating our ultimate Performance Day.

All day.

Every day.

OUR STORY

ath-lete. n. 1. one who participates in competitive sports. 2. a person who is trained or skilled in exercises, sports, tactics, or games requiring physical strength, agility, or stamina.

Athletes' Performance, the company my wife, Amy, and I started in 1999, is a global leader in human performance, and we say that with the utmost humility and responsibility. My colleagues and I are eager to support the world's highest performers, leaving no ethical stone unturned to help them achieve new levels of success.

You don't have to take my word for that. Our training centers in the United States, as well as our staff working around the globe, have had an impact on every sport imaginable. Though we're perhaps best known for our work in soccer, American football, and baseball, our athletes have received most every accolade in sports.

Our high-performance system goes beyond the toughest arenas of sport to the toughest environments anywhere. We have worked with US Special Operations, the world's most elite fighting forces, to meet their needs both home and abroad so they produce results regardless of where they are deployed. We've worked with other tactical athletes, including law enforcement and other first responders, to help them perform at the highest levels.

Whether in sports, in the military, or with first responders, we've demonstrated to the world's elite how they can do their jobs better at the highest global level, day in and day out. We apply the same thought process of doing things differently to the world's leading corporations, who also deeply value their human capital, helping them to generate greater efficiency and quality of life for their teams.

We've partnered with the likes of Intel, Walgreens, Sheraton Hotels and Resorts, LinkedIn, and other leading companies to set new standards in corporate wellness and employee productivity.

If you've followed one of our previous books or the programs on our CorePerformance.com website, some of the material in this book might sound familiar. Our organization of Mindset, Nutrition, Movement, and Recovery can be found in these pages.

Since writing this book, we've unified our two communities of Athletes' Performance and Core Performance into one united brand name, EXOS. At the time this book went to press, we were just beginning the transition to our new brand name, so you'll find references to EXOS, Athletes' Performance, and Core Performance in this book.

Our brand is for anyone willing to accept the challenge of taking his or her performance to the highest level possible. This book, however, is meant for what we call our founding audience: the elite performers and those who strive to be elite performers, the same folks who walk through the doors of our Athletes' Performance training centers.

This program is for the elite athlete in sport and elite tactical athletes, which is to say the elite military and first responders such as firefighters, police, and paramedics. It's for dedicated performers who are accountable to those they serve and protect. We have had the honor to support some of these agencies. We hope that this book serves you well since your communities are underfunded and underappreciated.

If you've followed the Core Performance system and are looking to perform at an even higher level, we're proud and grateful that you've turned to us again. You will, however, find it much more challenging, and ultimately more rewarding, to embrace the concept of *Every Day Is Game Day*.

That's because we've pushed ourselves to higher levels of performance every year since our founding in 1999. When the top teams and organizations in sport, let alone the US Department of Defense, turn to us to maximize their human capital, we know we must be at our highest level of performance every day. That's what drives our culture at EXOS.

We don't just teach this culture; we live it.

We've taken the same science we use to help our EXOS family operate at the highest level and have continued to upgrade it based on research and feedback from clients. We're always testing, learning, and applying this research to improve our system in the most responsible and ethical ways for our athletes and organizations.

When we talk about elite performers, it's not just about high-profile athletes in the field. It's also about the management and decision makers who must be on their A-games as well. They're making decisions on how to apply limited resources of human capital to fight the fight and accomplish goals in combat, business, and sport.

The US Department of Defense and top sports teams spend millions on their human capital. An elite tactical athlete is not easily replaced. Nor is a top player in the National Football League or Major League Baseball. The majority of injuries in sport, in the military, and among first responders, however, are non-deployment, non-game injuries. The injuries occur through inadequate training and often are driven by poor lifestyle choices. When an organization is missing elite performers, whether in the military, business, or sport, the implications can be devastating.

The value of these elite individuals is so high that you have to be able to keep them on the field of play competing at the highest level for as long as possible.

That's our job, our shared responsibility.

That's also our promise to you for making this commitment. This book isn't about your becoming better at training in the sport of fitness. It's about your becoming the best at what you're uniquely positioned to do.

For no matter what your occupation, goals, or interests, you have the potential to be an elite performer.

Our mission here, just as it is at all our EXOS locations around the world, is to help you become one.

HIGH-PERFORMANCE DNA

We're the sum of our behaviors. Ninety percent of our actions are driven by habits, whether positive or negative. Who we are today physically, emotionally, mentally, professionally, and financially is a reflection of our behaviors and the choices we've made to this point.

If you've fallen short in one of these areas—and who among us has not to some degree?—the reason is that you have not installed what we call the "high-performance DNA" necessary to drive your daily actions. You won't literally change your DNA, but it might seem that way, since you can dramatically change both your body and your performance if you're willing to do the work.

As we mentioned earlier, your best isn't good enough. You must continually strive to upgrade your system.

The goal is to have a longer and more productive career. We work with players in the National Football League, where the average career is 3.7 years. The catch-22 is that it often takes players three seasons to master the league's complex schemes and systems. Unfortunately for many, the physical toll ends their careers just as they're reaching this sweet spot of performance.

Those who have upgraded their systems, creating this new normal, can stay in the NFL for eight to ten seasons—or even longer—and still have some of the best years of their careers. By improving their performance and decreasing risk of injury, they receive huge returns on their investments of time working this system.

The same is true with Special Operations forces. Many of these tactical athletes bear the cost physically after serving our country through many missions, even though above the neck they continue to master the skill sets, language, and rituals necessary not just to stay alive, but also to execute operations. They bear this cost physically because they've sustained multiple injuries in combat and training. With this system, they can continue this vital role supporting our country into their forties and beyond.

No matter what your field, the goal should be to extend this priceless period in which your knowledge and experience can be best deployed. For too many people in all walks of life, not just the dangerous worlds of the military, first responders, and the NFL, they fail to maximize these high-performance, high-earning years because they do not have a system in place to reduce the potential of injury and physical deterioration.

This isn't a luxury or an option. If you don't have high-performance DNA in the military, you're dead, and perhaps also responsible for the deaths of others. If you don't have it in sports, you're more likely to be injured, underperforming, and unemployed. If you don't have it in the cutthroat world of business, you're bankrupt and financially ruined.

High performers look at the world differently. They know time is precious, but are willing to invest small amounts in a precise, disciplined way to minimize the risk of injury and maximize return on investment. It's no different from investing financially.

One example: A proper ten-minute warm-up before a training session aggregates into roughly forty-eight hours of training a year. (That's ten minutes per day, five or six days a week.) Yet that investment of time will pay huge dividends. This ten minutes, which in this program includes what we call Pillar Preparation and Movement Preparation, will make your workouts far more effective and reduce the risk of injury both during that session and long term.

Your sleep ritual, a topic we'll discuss later, is another daily ten-minute commitment that produces huge benefits. By implementing simple changes in your sleep ritual, you will change your hormonal profile over the course of a year.

High performers look for these windows of opportunity over the course of their days. Let's say you're stuck in traffic, a presentation, or a meeting. Take that opportunity to reset your posture and go through breathing techniques that will energize you when you might otherwise feel groggy.

When it comes to training, high performers know that what happens in the gym or on the practice field is a small part of the equation. We can upgrade performance in so many other ways throughout the day in smaller chunks of time. Best of all, it's integrated into our routines, which become our subconscious habits.

We're effectively training ourselves across a platform for high performance.

The four pillars of that platform are Mindset, Nutrition, Movement, and Recovery. Since every day is game day, you must:

Prepare for It. (Mindset)
Fuel for It. (Nutrition)
Train for It. (Movement)
Rest for It. (Recovery)

MINDSET: High performers have a focused mindset that minimizes distraction. That's increasingly challenging in the digital age. They understand their unique individual goals and their "IT," the thing that drives them most, which we'll establish early in this book. Most of all, they're constantly looking for ways to be smarter and more efficient in everything they do. Without a proper mindset 24/7, high performance is impossible.

NUTRITION: Food is fuel for the body and brain. It's not about diets or obsessing about portions of carbohydrate, protein, and fats. It's cutting through the latest diet marketing hype and nonsense and consuming what fuels you properly. Period. Proper fueling and hydration strategies improve cognition, energy, and endurance to maximize performance. When it comes to fueling, high performers constantly plan to ensure they will have the proper fuel available to achieve their IT.

MOVEMENT: High performers move effectively and efficiently through their professional requirements, as well as physically through all three planes of motion. Their bodies exhibit the mobility, stability, and power that nature intended. By working to counteract the effects of a sedentary society that has us hunched over computers and steering wheels much of the day, they create lean, powerful physiques that serve as the vehicles for professional and personal success.

RECOVERY: Growth happens during rest. It's when the mind and body repair, recharge, and upgrade. Recovery strategies must be employed throughout your day, week, month, and year. Yet they're often ignored in our fast-paced culture, where people assume the answer is working longer and harder. High performers know that it's about working more efficiently, prioritizing recovery, and using it to further fuel successes.

If you've followed the Core Performance program, the four-pronged Mindset-Nutrition-Movement-Recovery strategy will sound familiar. But make no mistake: EXOS is a 24/7 system for high performance that will permeate every aspect of your existence.

It starts with the integration of the system. Recovery is a Mindset. Movement is supported by Nutrition and vice versa. Nutrition and Movement support Recovery. And the high-performance Mindset is a thread woven throughout the entire program. These are not stand-alone pillars—Mindset, Nutrition, Movement, and Recovery—but rather the integrated strands of being a high performer.

We all have the same twenty-four hours a day. The quality of how we execute this program determines whether or not we're high performers.

When we do so, we achieve the Performance Day.

THE PERFORMANCE DAY

There are countless fitness and nutrition books. We've written five of them that we daresay are pretty damned good, respected by our peers and passionate performers.

The shortcoming with those books, including our own, is that they are meant for those whose professions and lifestyles do not require a 24/7 commitment. You're not held accountable for literally your entire day. Your success or failure is graded almost exclusively on how well you follow a workout and nutrition program. For most people, making a commitment to such a program produces massive change, which is a wonderful thing.

For an elite performer, it's not enough.

The difference for our clients and with this book is the concept of the Performance Day. Within EXOS we've often referred to this as the "perfect day." Unfortunately, many outside our community think of a perfect day in terms of lounging on a white-sand beach with a loved one, sipping frozen adult beverages while being caressed by warm ocean breezes.

The Performance Day is where champions are made. It's the idea that we're making a 24/7 commitment to being high performers across Mindset, Nutrition, Movement, and Recovery from the moment we wake up until the time we go to bed. Plus, since we're following proper sleep rituals, the Performance Day extends to the time we're asleep.

In this program, you will create *your* Performance Day from when you wake up until you go to bed. Ninety percent of our actions run in our subconscious, so we have to work hard to upgrade our daily rituals.

By doing that, you will have an actionable way to keep score of your daily performance. You'll create what we call an achiever mindset, the mindset of those who want to be even better tomorrow than they are today.

In this program, we're going to grade ourselves every day. There's a tendency to think professional athletes get graded only on game day. In reality, they're graded every day in practice. Whether they get an opportunity to compete on game day depends on how they perform during that preparation.

For most of us, there's not even that subtle distinction between the importance of practice and game day. Every Day Is Game Day. There is no dress rehearsal. You have to hit all targets and goals every day.

In this program, we'll grade ourselves on training (Movement) and fueling (Nutrition). But we'll also grade our performance starting with our morning ritual, ending with our evening routines, and including how we positioned ourselves for an improved tomorrow. When we can do that for a twenty-four-hour cycle, we've achieved the Performance Day.

We're not asking you to be perfect. The goal is to make the best decisions possible out of every given situation. If you improve your environment in terms of Mindset, Nutrition, Movement, and Recovery, you'll be in a better position to make effective decisions.

You are a function of your behaviors, which are driven by choices. Eighty percent is the new 100 percent. If you can be 80 percent successful in your choices 100 percent of the time, that's effective.

Nobody is confident of hitting 100 percent 100 percent of the time. But you can be confident of reaching 80 percent 100 percent of the time.

When you've done that, you've achieved a sustainable performance system, a Performance Day.

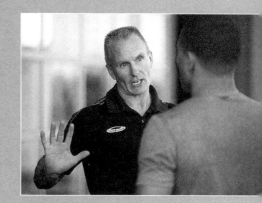

1 | PREPARE FOR IT

Athletes' Performance Mindset

WHAT IS THE ONE THING CALLING YOU TO ACTION RIGHT NOW? ALL OF US HAVE that one thing that drives us, the motivation to get out of bed in the morning. Perhaps it's a number of things, but chances are that even then they're tied to one driving force that calls you to be an elite performer.

So what is it? What is your "IT"?

At EXOS, we define IT as our purpose. Defining that purpose, that IT, dictates your performance game plan.

Once we have identified IT, we can Prepare for It, Fuel for It, Train for It, and Rest for It. The key is not to think of IT as a goal or end, but rather as a mantra, a statement that summarizes who you are, what drives you, and where you want to be.

That simple IT statement, as little as five words, will guide every decision and action over the course of your Performance Day. It provides the context for everything you do or choose not to do.

In just a moment, we'll go through a brief exercise to create your IT statement. It should be a solo effort. Don't enlist help from anyone, even a significant other who might know you better than you think you know yourself.

After all, you are the expert in everything "you." You know best how *you* have succeeded and where things haven't worked out. This is a process to help inspire the choices you make in life, tapping into that expertise to help you develop purpose in everything *you* do. You will turn to this IT statement several times a day throughout this program.

This IT statement will be the driver of your decisions and habits across the Athletes' Performance system of Mindset, Nutrition, Movement, and Recovery. Without the best foods, the brain will not have the energy or nutrients it needs to operate properly. Without Recovery, it can't think differently. Without increasingly challenging Movement, the critical circuits in the brain will not be activated to promote new thinking. Finally, without adapting this Mindset, your old thoughts will not let go to allow new ones to be created.

In other words, without adopting the integrated approach of Mindset, Nutrition, Movement, and Recovery, you won't create the proper brain environment to have a chance to become a high performer. Mind over matter is not enough.

This IT Illuminator process is designed as a guideline to align your motivations with your behavior to reflect what is most important. Taking fifteen minutes to go through the exercise defines what is important and builds the confidence to live in alignment with your IT. It creates a context to view your daily decisions so that your actions reflect what you're trying to achieve.

Your IT statement could revolve around family, career, or health. It doesn't matter as long as you dig deep enough to get at the core of what is most important. If you're like some of our clients who face life-and-death decisions daily, you might need two IT statements: one for "home" and one for "away."

Once you have created this IT statement, repeat it several times a day. It will be part of your morning and evening rituals. You could print it out and place it on your nightstand, bathroom mirror, refrigerator, or desk. Perhaps you will take a favorite photo and emblazon the IT statement onto it. Don't just repeat it to yourself, though. Visualize the benefits of living your life that way. Writing just a key word from it on your wrist before a big event helps you quickly visualize why you are there, especially in critical moments.

Why is this IT statement so important? Our minds operate in three ways. There's the conscious process, the subconscious process, and the creative non-conscious process. It is through these areas that we create and maintain a vision of ourselves, which, for better or for worse, dictates our corresponding "realities." If we continue to see ourselves in a negative light, our subconscious will cause our performances to be consistent with our current image of truth and reality. That translates into negative performance. On the other hand, a more positive view will translate into positive performance, as the deeply held self-image responds to your positivity.

Since the Athletes' Performance program is an integrated system, it will do us little good to install the right habits across our Movement, Nutrition, and Recovery if we don't improve our Mindset. In fact, it becomes much more difficult to do so if we don't have that driving force, that IT statement, to guide our actions.

Mindset is where we have an opportunity to influence ourselves twenty-four hours a day. Our current reality will define our future only if we allow it. World-class athletes remain that way as long as they maintain world-class habits. Like-wise, people who struggle in specific areas continue to struggle because of their habits and decisions.

Decisions are a result of the repetition of negative or positive actions and thoughts. Through the IT Illuminator process, we will define what's most important to us, create this anchor IT statement, and reinforce its power by looking at the advantages and disadvantages to living (or not living) along those lines.

The reason this is so important for high achievers is that you need to find a driving force that goes far beyond the scope of diet and exercise books. You must be guided by a far deeper reason—and you are, whether you realize it or not—than just wanting to pack on ten pounds of muscle or lose twenty pounds of fat. That's the breakthrough. When you're able to govern all of your daily actions and deci-sions by whether they align with this IT statement, that's when you tap into the power of being a high achiever.

Let's discover this IT statement by going through the following exercise. From the words on the chart on page 16, write down the ten that jump out as most valu-able and meaningful to you at this moment in your life. You don't have to pick one from each category; you could have multiple from one category and none from

IT Iluminator

Write down ten words that are meaningful to you. Then circle the three that are most meaningful to you right now.

1.

2.

3.

4.

5.

6.

7.

8.

9.

10.

Create a statement that tells a story about living your life in the best way possible.

Enter your IT Statement here.

Physical Performance	Pain	Appearance
Endurance	Relief	Lean
Fitness	Pain-Free	Choice
Strength	Freedom	Comfort
Power	Activity	Confidence
Speed	Movement	Attractiveness
Resilience	Function	Youthfulness
Personal Best	Prevention	Tone
Health	**Relationships**	**Energy**
Vitality	Family	Energy
Longevity	Commitment	Empowerment
Health	Responsibility	Restful
Quality of Life	Giving	Focus
Feel Alive	Connection	Alertness
Aging	Support	Vitality
Spirituality	Presence	Enthusiasm
Emotional Well-being	**Work Performance**	**Challenge (New Things)**
Balance	Focus	Evolve
Presence	Efficiency	Try
Motivation	Productivity	Open
Calmness	Communication	Exciting
Happiness	Creativity	Accomplish
Contentment	Success	Challenge
Optimism	Organization	Goal

others. If you wish to add a word to a particular category to make it fit yourself better, feel free to do so.

This is a uniquely individual process, but perhaps it would help to use an example. Let's say we have a thirty-nine-year-old married father of two. He's a high achiever, a leader in his field, an accomplished athlete by any definition. We'll call him John.

John chose one word from each of the nine categories but, again, feel free to choose whichever ten words best fit you; you can pick multiple words from the same category. Here are the words John chose: Strength (Physical Performance), Freedom (Pain), Lean (Appearance), Quality of Life (Health), Family (Relationships), Focus (Energy), Optimism (Emotional Well-being), Success (Work Performance), Evolve (Challenge). John added his own word—Prolific—to round out his ten.

From the ten words you chose, circle the three that are the most meaningful to you right now. The three words should reflect what is important in your life.

John chose Focus, Family, and Freedom. His reasoning was that Family is the most important aspect of his life; Focus gives him energy (and also was listed under Work Performance, so it had a two-pronged meaning for him); and Freedom from pain, as listed in this context, is important. But John also thought of Freedom in terms of the ability for himself and his family to have the opportunities to experience everything life has to offer.

Next, using these three words, create a statement that tells a story about living your life in the best way possible. Try to steer the statement toward a vision of what your life will become rather than what specifically you will do to get there.

John managed to do both with his statement. He wrote, *I will provide Freedom for my Family to acquire meaningful experiences together by maintaining Focus to take advantage of opportunities.* His reasoning was that if he stayed *focused* on providing *freedom* for his *family*, all of his daily actions would be driven by a vision of giving himself and his family all of the wonderful opportunities in life.

In the grid on page 18 there are four boxes. Let's go back to the vision of your ideal life you created with the three words you circled. Think about all the disadvantages to *not* living in alignment with your description of your best life identified in the previous steps and write them down in the top left box.

For John, this was simple, though a bit scary. If he did not rediscover his focus at work and in the rest of his life, he would not be able to provide the freedom and opportunities for himself and his family. He considered what impact that might have on the lives of his children and even his marriage. He thought of his recent

Intention Statement:

DISADVANTAGES

ADVANTAGES

NOT LIVING IN ALIGNMENT

LIVING IN ALIGNMENT

athletic performance and how that had gone downhill. He marveled at how poorly he was eating and how infrequently he was training and how that would impact his quality of life down the road, or even how long that road would be. It was not a pretty picture.

Now think about all the advantages of *not* living in alignment with your description of your best life and write them down in the box at the top right of the same grid.

John struggled to come up with anything to write in this box. He shrugged, figuring there was a sort of comfort level in the status quo. His family seemed relatively happy at the moment, and he felt somewhat accomplished at work, though he was mistaking being busy for being productive. He knew such a good-but-not-great situation was not sustainable and that something was going to give. Either he was going to keep toiling harder and less efficiently at work, taking more time away from his family, or he might become so inefficient that his career would suffer. Neither option was attractive.

After ten minutes, John's "advantages" box remained nearly empty. Clearly there was little advantage to *not* living with his description of his best life.

Next, think about all the disadvantages of living in alignment with your description of your best life and write them down in the box at the bottom left of the grid.

John could not come up with much to write in this square, either. He figured the process of getting refocused and going all in with the Athletes' Performance program from a Mindset, Nutrition, Movement, and Recovery standpoint might require an uncomfortable transition period. He would need to overhaul his nutrition, reestablish some good habits around movement, and commit to recovery rituals every day, week, month, and year. But that seemed like a small price to pay.

Think about all the advantages of living in alignment with your description of your best life and write them down in the box at the bottom right.

This time, the words flowed quickly for John. He thought of a future where his children had the opportunities to flourish and he and his wife could enjoy all of the things they'd talked about for years. He thought back to when his career and athletic performance were at their peaks and realized that he should—and could—establish a new benchmark for success. He did not have to settle for the status quo and could break out of his current vicious cycle that slowly was robbing him of his most precious commodity: time.

I will provide Freedom for my Family to acquire meaningful experiences to-gether by maintaining Focus to take advantage of opportunities.

Take a look at the upper left and bottom right boxes. If you don't live your life in alignment with the statement you just wrote using your three words, the con-trast between the life you want and the one you might have could be large. With a few simple changes moving forward, you can ensure that the bottom right becomes your actual life in the future.

Now take a look at the upper right and bottom left boxes. These boxes rep-resent your barriers to living your ideal life: bad habits in the upper right, and automatic, nonconscious excuses and perceptions in the bottom left.

Finally, take a look back at everything you've written. Study it and take a mo-ment to soak it all in. Now, using five words or less, create your IT statement to capture all of the emotion, intent, purpose, and power of what you've written.

Focus was a key word for John. It tied him to his broader vision of providing freedom and opportunity for his family. But it also had a more practical application. In the age of digital distraction, he found it challenging to keep from constantly checking his digital devices and immediately dealing with everyone who wanted a piece of his time. Social media, texts, and instant messages all took chunks of his time and his attention. As a result, he often felt busy but not like he was getting a lot done. In fact, he felt constantly behind on work. His time management, for years a strength, was now a weakness. His nutrition and athletic performance also suffered.

John figured if he could remain focused on family freedom, he could make his vision a reality.

Thinking about everything he had put down on paper and the intent behind it, John came up with his five-word IT statement: *Stay Focused For Family Freedom.*

The key word in John's IT statement was *For.* Had he gone with "Stay Focused *On* Family Freedom," the statement would have been one-dimensional and less powerful. By going with *For,* it became both a vision and an action statement. He even capitalized *For,* even though it technically was not grammatically correct, to emphasize its importance. (John even could have gone with "Stay Focused *Four* Family Freedom," a reference to the four pillars of the Athletes' Performance pro-gram: Mindset, Nutrition, Movement, and Recovery.)

Your vision, your IT statement, no doubt will be much different from John's. That's important, because this needs to be a personalized process. Those who make their own arguments for why they want to change their unhealthy behaviors

John's IT lluminator

Write down ten words that are meaningful to you. Then circle the three that are most meaningful to you right now.

1. Strength
2. (Freedom)
3. Lean
4. Quality of Life
5. (Family)
6. (Focus)
7. Optimism
8. Success
9. Evolve
10. Prolific

Create a statement that tells a story about living your life in the best way possible.

I will provide Freedom for my Family to acquire meaningful experiences together by maintaining Focus to take advantage of opportunities.

Enter your IT Statement here.

Stay Focused For Family Freedom.

Physical Performance	Pain	Appearance
Endurance	Relief	Lean
Fitness	Pain-Free	Choice
Strength	Freedom	Comfort
Power	Activity	Confidence
Speed	Movement	Attractiveness
Resilience	Function	Youthfulness
Personal Best	Prevention	Tone
Health	**Relationships**	**Energy**
Vitality	Family	Energy
Longevity	Commitment	Empowerment
Health	Responsibility	Restful
Quality of Life	Giving	Focus
Feel Alive	Connection	Alertness
Aging	Support	Vitality
Spirituality	Presence	Enthusiasm
Emotional Well-being	**Work Performance**	**Challenge (New Things)**
Balance	Focus	Evolve
Presence	Efficiency	Try
Motivation	Productivity	Open
Calmness	Communication	Exciting
Happiness	Creativity	Accomplish
Contentment	Success	Challenge
Optimism	Organization	Goal

inevitably do so. We are more likely to believe what comes out of our own mouths than from experts', as the arguments we come up with are the most compelling for establishing importance, confidence, and readiness.

People don't mind change, which is good since high performers recognize that change is the only constant, but they hate being told what to do. People like to choose, and the purpose of the exercise is to help you choose from this menu of descriptive words to form a statement that's relevant on a personal level.

When people are at Point A in their life and don't see the need for a Point B, they stay as they are. When people are at Point A in their life and see a Point B that they think is better, they change. When people are at Point A in their life and see a Point B, which they think is better but perceive it to be too difficult to manage, they lose motivation to change and enter a state of ambivalence (*I want it but it's all too hard!* Or *I can't see myself doing that!*).

Does your IT statement describe your motivation in life right now? If not, go back and try again. Remember that you are not doing this for a twelve-week fitness program. You are learning the science and creating your system of sustainable performance for the rest of your life.

YOUR PERFORMANCE DAY
An Around-the-Clock Look

Now that you've defined your IT statement to power everything you do, let's create a game plan to achieve it, starting with your Performance Day. We will break down Nutrition, Movement, and Recovery in depth later, but for now let's take a quick around-the-clock look.

Tomorrow's success starts today. Since your day begins literally at midnight, sleep is a powerful part of your Performance Day and why we will build around it. What follows are not suggestions or a best-case scenario. This is what you *must* achieve, day in and day out, to instill yourself with the high-performance mindset.

MORNING RITUAL

You're actually most in control of your day during this time frame. It sets the tone for your success. Think of your morning and evening rituals as two bookends that you have full control over. Actually, as you'll discover in this program, it's possible to have more control over most of your day than you think, especially once you have these strong bookends in place. There's a high degree of chaos in between. The goal is to make the best decisions during those periods.

MINDSET: Upon waking, take a minute to give thanks for family, friends, career, and everything that's right with your life. Consider how your efforts today will elevate others. Visualize this upcoming Performance Day, the tasks at hand, and how you will accomplish them. Ponder the vision for who you are becoming and how you will navigate the day at the highest level. Take a few moments to visualize the benefits of living your IT statement. You could keep a printout of it on your nightstand, but presumably you'll have it memorized. Our friend John from the previous section will repeat *Stay Focused For Family Freedom*. Repeat your IT statement periodically throughout the morning ritual, visualizing the benefits of living it.

MOVEMENT: Your body has been at rest, which is a good thing, but we must get your fascia moving. Fascia are the connective tissues running from the top of your head to the bottom of your feet and into every cell of your body; they organize your powerful muscles. We can do this through what we call Movement Prep exercises (see pages 69–70). We also want to engage in some soft tissue work, such as rolling on a hard foam roller (see pages 277–282) or by using a massage stick (see pages 283–285).

NUTRITION: Though you might not feel thirsty, you're dehydrated after sleep. Drink 16 ounces of water upon waking. You should place a glass of water on your nightstand or bathroom sink before going to sleep (and drink from it during the night if you awaken).

As for breakfast, it's not just a cliché: It is the most important meal of the day. Actually, your postworkout fueling is more important—more on that in a moment—but breakfast is a strong second. There's no excuse for skipping breakfast, and it's important that you break the fast that started when you went to dinner by eating within thirty minutes of waking.

Breakfast boosts metabolism, fuels the brain, and provides energy. Consider drinking breakfast in the form of a nutrition-dense smoothie. Or eat something simple, such as whole grain toast with natural peanut butter, low-fat Greek yogurt, and a banana. Or try oatmeal with berries, almonds, and a hard-boiled egg. Another good option is an English muffin with scrambled eggs and avocado with 100 percent fruit juice. Whatever you choose, your breakfast should include high-fiber carbohydrates, lean protein, healthy fats, and color coming from fruits and vegetables.

Morning Ritual Summary

Mindset
Visualize Performance Day
Repeat IT statement and visualize
   benefits of living it

Movement
Movement Prep
Soft tissue massage

Nutrition
Drink 16 ounces of water
Breakfast or preworkout fueling
Multivitamin/fish oil

Recovery
Targeted breathing

Working out first thing in the morning is the best time for many people. You've accomplished something while most are asleep and avoided the potential of something interfering with your training session later in the day. We'll provide pre- and postworkout nutrition options shortly.

This also is an ideal time to consume a multivitamin and some fish oil. Multivitamins cover any deficiencies your diet might be lacking. Fish oil provides powerful omega-3 fatty acids, which have anti-inflammatory properties, regulate blood sugar, and are essential for good cardiovascular health and mental clarity.

RECOVERY: Even though you just woke up, it's still time to recover. Take this time to extend your breath. Breathe in through your nose for six counts, hold for four counts, and breathe out through your mouth for ten counts. This extended breath out slows your breathing, reduces stress, and induces calmness. Repeat this pattern ten times to calm your nervous system and decrease cortisol production. This targeted breathing can be done during the Mindset or Movement portions of your morning ritual.

LATE MORNING RITUAL

There's a tendency to view the part of the day between breakfast and lunch as a time to put your head down and simply hammer through tasks, regardless of your profession or athletic career. As a high performer, however, you still must incorporate the pattern of Mindset-Nutrition-Movement-Recovery throughout the late morning hours. Here's how:

MINDSET: As you leave home—or even if you operate out of home—visualize the performance athlete you want to be. Consider how you will perform the next few hours. Repeat your IT statement several times and visualize the benefits of living it.

NUTRITION: There are likely five to seven hours between your breakfast and lunch. Eating smaller meals more often controls appetite and regulates blood sugar. It improves concentration, eliminates mood swings and overeating, and maintains muscle mass. Have a midmorning fueling that includes a combination of colorful high-fiber carbs, protein, and fat.

Try fruit, veggies, nuts, sunflower seeds, or beef jerky. If you have access to a blender or shaker bottle, a shake or smoothie consisting of fruit and whey protein also is a good option. Note that we use the word *fuel*, never *snack*. Snacking is synonymous with junk food, or at least what you give the dog. Fuel powers your brain and body for success.

By having this midmorning fueling, you'll find you won't need your typical lunch. It likely will be smaller, but should again consist of high-fiber carbs, lean protein, healthy fats, and color.

Wherever your morning takes you—or even if you remain at home—continue to drink water. Even minor dehydration impairs concentration, coordination, and reaction time. Drink ½ to 1 ounce of water per pound of body weight per day to maintain hydration.

MOVEMENT/RECOVERY: It can be difficult to maintain good posture while spending a chunk of your day sitting down, whether driving, receiving briefings,

Your Performance Day Sample Meals

TIME—MEAL

7 a.m.—Oatmeal, berries, 2 eggs, 2 tablespoons flaxseeds

9:15 a.m.—Preworkout shooter

11:15 a.m.—Postworkout shake

12:15 p.m.—Turkey sandwich on 100 percent whole wheat bread with 6 ounces turkey, avocado, and piled with other vegetables, along with a spinach salad with olive oil and vinegar dressing

3 p.m.—Apple with ¼ cup nuts

6 p.m.—5 ounces grilled salmon, ½ cup whole wheat couscous, steamed asparagus drizzled with olive oil and lemon after cooking

9:30 p.m.—1 cup low-fat cottage cheese and ½ cup berries

Late Morning Ritual Summary

Mindset
Visualize Performance Day
Repeat IT statement and visualize
   benefits of living it

Movement
Movement break
Posture check

Nutrition
Midmorning fueling and lunch
Hydrate (rate of ½ to 1 ounce
   per pound per day)

Recovery
Trigger point therapy

or sitting in meetings. That's why it's important to check your posture a couple times each morning. Are your shoulder blades pulled back and down? Is your chest elevated? Are you "sitting tall"?

Even if you're stuck in a seated position, you still can use this time productively. Work on one set of ten anchor breaths, inhaling for up to six seconds, holding for four seconds, and exhaling for eight to ten seconds.

Most people make it a point on long flights to get up and walk around. So why do most of us not rise from our meetings for hours unless nature calls? Take periodic five-minute breaks and do some simple Movement Prep (see pages 69–70). These movements counteract the effects of the modern sedentary society, which are to round our shoulders, lock our hips, and weaken our cores.

Keep a tennis ball under your desk. While standing or sitting, slip off your shoe and roll your foot back and forth over the tennis ball, applying pressure to the arch of your foot. This trigger point therapy will help relieve chronic foot pain and fascial tightness. According to Eastern medicine, this process also improves overall health.

AFTERNOON RITUAL

The morning hours tend to be the most productive ones. But the afternoon is the key to your Performance Day. High school and college athletes train during the mid- to late-afternoon hours. This isn't just for scheduling purposes; studies suggest these are the most effective times for physical activity. Even if your schedule makes training at this point impossible, there still are things you must do to stay on track toward your Performance Day.

Afternoon Ritual Summary

Mindset
Quick check on progress of daily goals
Repeat IT statement and visualize
    benefits of living it

Movement
Movement break
Posture check

Nutrition
Midafternoon fueling
Maintain hydration goals

Recovery
Midafternoon nap

MINDSET: After lunch, review your day. Are you on track to reach your goals? Are you following the vision you set for the day earlier? Repeat your IT statement several times and visualize the benefits of living it. Have your actions thus far supported that statement? In other words, are your actions bringing IT to life?

NUTRITION: Assuming lunch falls between twelve and one and dinner between six and seven, the three-to-four-p.m. hour is the perfect time for a light fueling to keep your metabolism firing and your mind sharp. Good options to stash in a desk drawer include nuts, beef/turkey jerky, meal replacement bars, and apples. As always, make it a balance of carbs, lean protein, healthy fats, and color.

Don't let up on hydration. You should be on at least your second bottle of water, not including the water you had at breakfast, lunch, and to wash down your midmorning fuel.

MOVEMENT: Nobody would sit through all-day meetings or film sessions without taking at least one ten-minute break (for reasons other than nature calling). So why deprive yourself when it's just you? Take a few minutes and go for a walk, do some Movement Prep exercises, and reset your posture to offset the effects of sitting hunched over for any period of time. If you're leading a group, create a performance culture by calling your colleagues to take action accordingly.

RECOVERY: Some of the busiest, most noteworthy leaders in history have benefited from short fifteen- to twenty-minute midafternoon naps. So there's no reason you can't find the time. Taking a brief break and clearing your mind has been shown to greatly enhance your creativity later in the day. Don't worry if you don't fall asleep; just closing your eyes and relaxing will be refreshing. Find a dark,

Pre- and Postworkout Fueling

You never want to be deprived of nutrients, especially when you work out. Eat something before you train, even if it's just half an apple with a handful of nuts, a slice of whole wheat toast with natural peanut butter, yogurt, or a preworkout "shooter" consisting of a glass of watered-down orange juice with a scoop of whey protein.

You *must* eat within thirty minutes after training, preferably within ten. Don't waste your workout. When you've finished training, your cells are wide open and screaming for nutrients. The quickest and easiest way to replenish them is with a postworkout recovery shake made with a protein powder (or supplement), such as EAS Recovery Protein. By having a shake right after your workout, you stop the stress hormone cortisol secretion and start the positive hormones and nutrients to expedite the recovery process and maximize lean muscle growth. If you go through the effort to train and move your body and don't take measures to repair it, you've wasted your workout. Whoever recovers the quickest and most effectively has a competitive advantage.

quiet place and close the door so you will not be disturbed. Set a timer so you don't stress about oversleeping.

EVENING RITUAL

The evening is no time to let up on the gas on your Performance Day. In fact, Recovery strategies become even more important, especially as you transition into the sleep ritual period.

MINDSET: If you're returning home from work and/or training, take a few moments to transition mentally in the car. Leave work in the car, figuratively speaking. Visualize living your IT and its benefits. Once inside your home, seek out loved ones and greet them with hugs and kisses, don't talk about work. Next, change into more comfortable clothes. Not only is this good for recovery, it changes you into a Mindset of Recovery.

NUTRITION: Keep drinking water on your trip home. Chances are you didn't drink enough throughout the day. Not only that, but staying hydrated will keep you from overeating at dinner. Stop drinking a half hour or more before your meal.

Dinner should consist of lean protein, colorful fruits and vegetables, fiber-rich

Evening Ritual Summary

Mindset
Transition mentally from work to recovery
Repeat IT statement and visualize
benefits of living it

Movement/Recovery
Foam rolling and AIS or static stretching
Get off and elevate feet

Nutrition
Dinner and prebedtime fueling
Stay on track with hydration
goals

carbs, and healthy fats. Since you've been eating more frequent meals, your dinner likely will be smaller. It does not have to carry you over until breakfast. Have a light fueling fifteen to thirty minutes before bed. One option is a cup of low-fat cottage cheese and ½ cup of berries.

MOVEMENT/RECOVERY: Whether you've trained earlier in the day or just hours ago, power down with some foam rolling (see pages 277–282), Active Isolated Stretching (AIS), or static stretching. Get off your feet and elevate them above your heart if possible.

SLEEP RITUAL

Few people give any thought to a sleep ritual and the impact it has not only on sleep but also on their performance throughout the day. We'll discuss at length the importance of sleep in Recovery (pages 118–124), including the value of getting eight hours of sleep a night, but for now just understand that it's important to go through a sleep ritual to prepare your body and create the proper environment to get the most out of sleep.

If you've managed to hit all of these targets for twenty-four hours, you have achieved your Performance Day.

Sleep deeply.

One down and 364 to go.

Your Performance Day Checklist

Got eight hours of sleep

Completed morning ritual

Ate breakfast

Fueled midmorning

Completed midmorning posture check,
did five minutes of movement,
focused on breathing

Ate lunch

Fueled midafternoon

Completed a midafternoon
posture check, did five minutes
movement, and focused on
breathing

Took a nap or at least rested with feet up for
twenty minutes

Ate dinner

Fueled prebedtime

Followed sleep ritual

Completed planned training

Consumed adequate pretraining nutrition
(see page 48)

Hydrated adequately during training
(see pages 46–47)

Consumed postworkout nutrition within ten
minutes or ASAP

Reached adequate twenty-four-hour
hydration (see pages 45–46)

Fueling at a Glance

Include lean proteins, colorful fruits and
vegetables, high-fiber carbs, and fit fats

Breakfast: Whole grains, oatmeal, fruit, eggs,
almonds, avocado

Midmorning/midafternoon/prebedtime fuel:
meal replacement bar or shake, sandwich,
fruit, nuts, beef jerky

Lunch/dinner: lean meat, fish, veggies, fruit,
whole grain bread, whole wheat pasta,
brown rice

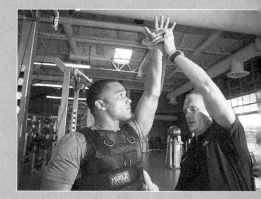

2 | FUEL FOR IT

Athletes' Performance Nutrition

NUTRITION NEED NOT BE COMPLICATED. IN FACT, LET'S TOSS OUT THE WORD *nutrition* and think in terms of fuel. We're fueling our bodies for high performance. We fuel to perform, fuel to recover, and fuel to win.

Our views of nutrition typically are shaped by the latest fad diets, popular ingredients, or some new "fact" jumped upon by the media. We've been left to figure out proper fueling for ourselves, navigating through the countless books and Web pages. This avalanche of information has left us in a state of paralysis, unable to make sense of all the conflicting advice.

Naturally, we want to perform our best in every situation. We want to have the energy needed to stay mentally focused and physically strong. We want to boost our immune system and speed the recovery process. Nutrition plays a critical role in all of our brains' and bodies' functions, yet most of us adjust the way we eat only to make a change in body composition. You cannot overstate the importance of proper fueling on your brain and cognition. How you eat impacts your brain's ability to function, perhaps the most important variable in performance.

At EXOS, when we present Nutrition 101 to the most elite athletes in the sports and tactical fields, there still are chuckles at the beginning of the lecture from those who ate pizza the night before or those consuming soda as we speak. By the end of the lecture, they realize that performance nutrition is not about focusing on carrots and celery sticks. The way the body is fueled makes or breaks your performance. Period.

You might not realize it because you don't know how great you can feel with proper fueling. The longer you consume foods that do not provide the proper fuel and nutrients, the more you cause inflammation and create an energy deficit. In fact, you're probably operating at such a deficit, relying on sugar and caffeine just to get through the day, that you've lost the energetic feeling that comes only from putting the proper nutrients, the ideal fuel, into your body.

Those nutrients do not magically appear; they must come from food. You need to look at your life, your day, and your meals and ask, "Am I making inspired choices with my fuel and hydration?"

Our society is overfed and undernourished. Each time you eat it is an opportunity to provide nutrients that produce stable energy, immune protection, general repair, cellular rejuvenation, and a decrease in inflammation.

When it comes to nutrition, are you leaving something on the table? From now on, think of nutrition and diet not as something to change your body composition. Instead, view nutrition as a process of making the most of every fueling opportunity—to fuel your Performance Day, to fuel your IT.

HOW TO EAT

You've probably never given much thought to building a meal. Hunger and personal tastes play a big role, but that's not what the motivation should be. The goal of nutrition is to provide the body with stable energy and sufficient nutrients to perform. So how do we do that? Before diving into a nutritional to-do list, let's take a look at what we believe to be important from a performance nutrition standpoint.

This is a model of how to fuel your performance. There's a tendency to debate

Color Your Plate

Heart Health	**Red**
	Cherries
	Beets
	Tomatoes

Circulation	**Blue/Purple**
	Blueberries
	Plums
	Eggplant

Immune System	**White**
	Garlic
	Onions
	Cauliflower

Musculature	**Green**
	Broccoli
	Spinach
	Kiwi

Brain Function	**Yellow**
	Pineapple
	Yellow peppers
	Star fruit

Skin and Eye Health	**Orange**
	Carrots
	Oranges
	Sweet potatoes

the merits of protein, carbs, and fats and the proper percentage of each. At EXOS, we replace that discussion by focusing on how we Fuel, Build, Protect, Prevent, and Hydrate.

Build your plate with the compass guiding your choices.

FUEL = minimally processed, high-fiber carbohydrates that provide sustainable energy

BUILD = lean proteins that provide the body the building blocks for repair and recovery

PROTECT = healthy fats that decrease inflammation and nourish the brain

PREVENT = colorful fruits and vegetables that provide the fiber, vitamins, minerals, and antioxidants needed for repair and immune function

HYDRATE = ½ to 1 ounce of water per pound of body weight per day

Getting It Done: Three Checkpoints

By the end of this section, you will have all the things necessary to upgrade your nutrition and create a new nutritional normal. These things will become second nature.

Checkpoint No. 1: Fuel Checkpoint. This is a real-time checklist to use while preparing meals and evaluating what you eat.

- Fuel
- Build
- Protect
- Prevent
- Hydrate

Did your meal or minimeal deliver in terms of fueling, building, protecting, preventing, and hydrating? Did you cover everything? To achieve your Performance Day, you have to nail this every time—or at least be at 80 percent or better 100 percent of the time.

Checkpoint No. 2: Fueling Strategy Checkpoint. There are fifteen key rules that we'll explain shortly. These are the keys to optimizing your nutritional success. The more consistently you follow these strategies, the better you will feel, the faster you will recover, and the closer you will be to knowing that you are doing everything you can to cover your bases from a nutritional standpoint.

Here are the strategies:

- View food as fuel
- Hit 80/20
- Fuel with minimally processed carbohydrates
- Power with lean proteins
- Eat fats that give back
- Eat the rainbow
- Eat breakfast every day
- Eat every three hours
- Meet your foundational hydration needs
- Stay hydrated during activity
- Fuel for your activity
- Stay fueled during your activity
- Refuel and rebuild after your workout
- Reach the proper level of foundational nutrition support
- Complement your training

Checkpoint No. 3: The Quick Nutrition Inventory. Once you better understand the five key nutrition principles, you can easily implement the inventory. At the end of each day, simply rank how well you did in the key areas on a scale of 1 to 5. You should aim for a 4 to 5 in each category.

Mindset	1	2	3	4	5
Eat Clean	1	2	3	4	5
Eat Often	1	2	3	4	5
Hydrate	1	2	3	4	5
Recover	1	2	3	4	5

- Mindset: Did you have a proactive approach to fueling today?
- Eat Clean: Did you choose mostly minimally processed, nutrient-dense food?
- Eat Often: Did you eat breakfast within the first thirty minutes of waking and eat every three hours after that?

- Hydrate: Did you drink half your body weight in ounces of water today? Did you lose less than 2 percent of your body weight during your activity?
- Recover: Did you properly fuel before, during, and after your activity? Did you take your multivitamin, fish oil, and other necessary nutritional complements (aka nutritional supplements)?

Bottom line: Before you eat, ask yourself if that meal or snack is the best choice to Fuel, Build, Protect, and Prevent.

Athletes' Performance Nutrition is not a diet. The word *diet*, by definition, refers to "food and drink regularly provided or consumed" or "habitual nourishment." Habitual nourishment—that's not a bad phrase. It's certainly better than the more popular definition of *diet*, which is to say short-term, unsustainable deprivation.

We do want to *habitually* consume the foods that *nourish* the body to give us the *fuel* to meet the challenges of daily life and perform at a world-class level.

Thus, food is fuel. When you have that energy and can perform better, you naturally perform *and* feel better. When you're able to make the correlation between how foods affect your body and energy level, you'll naturally gravitate toward them. You will stop eating and start fueling.

In short, you will "Fuel for It." *It* refers to success and high performance, but also that IT statement you crafted in the previous section. You're fueling to support that vision, that goal. In fact, use that IT statement as you're fueling, not just to reinforce your vision with the fuel you consume but also to make sure you fuel properly.

Remember our buddy John from the previous section? He repeats his IT statement and visualizes the benefits of living IT when he's putting together a high-performance meal: *Stay Focused For Family Freedom.* He knows his high-nutrient meal is fueling that vision. If he's in a less-than-ideal nutritional situation—on the road, out to dinner with friends at a restaurant with few quality options, etc.—he'll turn to that statement to help him make the best choice possible.

When it comes to fueling properly, there is a big misconception that you'll eat only bland, tasteless food. At EXOS, we have a world-class team of chefs that produces delicious meals packed with nutrients. Our athletes look forward to fueling in our cafe, often consuming all of their daily meals there.

One easy way to get a jump start on the week and save lots of time is to do all of your shopping on Saturdays or Sundays, which will help you plan meals for the week. This is a great way to be proactive about your choices. A little planning, preparing, and organizing of your environment will provide a huge return on your investment.

Here's the bottom line: When you don't give your body the fuel it needs, it becomes catabolic, drawing fuel from and depleting your lean muscle—the very thing you're working so hard to create. It's this lean muscle or "lean mass" that burns calories at a greater rate, even when you're resting. Unfortunately, this is the first thing your body turns to for fuel in this catabolic state.

When your body lacks the proper fuel to run or recover, its ability to take on the stress of daily life and training is substantially compromised, and it never has a chance to fully heal. This unbalanced state makes you more susceptible to sickness, fatigue, depression, inflammation, injury, and loss of motivation.

Even if you think you're fueling properly right now, I guarantee that the following pages will show you ways to fuel better and improve your performance. Nutrition should be used to enhance your energy and your performance in everything that you do.

You will Fuel your IT.

With that in mind, here are the simple yet powerful strategies for high-performance fueling.

Athletes' Performance Nutrition

1. Mindset
2. Eat Clean
3. Eat Often
4. Hydrate
5. Recover

1 | MINDSET

Eating is about fueling for high performance, not engaging in rich sensory culinary experiences. There's nothing wrong with that, of course, but think of those meals as special occasions. Your core day-to-day nutrition should be about fueling your body for success. Let's take a deeper look at those fifteen key strategies discussed earlier in the following sections:

1. FOOD = FUEL

Again, forget how you think of food. Instead, think of food in terms of what powers and sustains you.

2. THE 80/20 RULE

Background: Each meal and light fueling is an opportunity to fuel your body. Choose the foods that are best for you 80 percent of the time and incorporate some of those foods that may not be the best, but are your favorites, 20 percent of the time.

You're going to eat right at least 80 percent of the time and not beat yourself up about the other 20 percent. This isn't a dramatic departure from programs that recommend taking one day off a week and eating virtually anything you'd like. Eating "clean" six out of seven days represents 85.7 percent of the time. That's still a good target, but 80 percent is an acceptable benchmark.

Make It Happen: We are not, however, lowering the bar. This is not a relaxed approach to nutrition. Instead, it's a program of *mindful* eating as opposed to the typical *mindless* consumption of food.

> **Remember:** Hitting 80 percent, 100 percent of the time = Performance Day.

2 | EAT CLEAN

When it comes to eating clean, it's not just about washing your food thoroughly, though that's always important. Eating clean refers to making the best possible choice whenever you're selecting food.

Whole foods are the best choice, since they're unprocessed and unrefined, or at least processed and refined as little as possible prior to consumption. Whole foods typically do not contain added salt, sugar, or fat.

When grocery shopping, you'll usually find whole foods on the perimeter of the store. That's where you'll find the produce, meat and seafood, dairy, frozen foods, and other natural foods. These areas are refrigerated, which is no coincidence. The less processed a food is, the shorter its shelf life.

The middle aisles of a grocery store are the danger zones. Here you'll find snack foods, baking supplies, cereals, sodas, and condiments. Many of these processed foods can (and do) remain on shelves for months. Generally speaking, it's a good rule of thumb to work the perimeter.

Eating clean also means consuming the proper mix of carbs, proteins, and fats. All food is classified into these three nutrient groups, and if you neglect any of the three, you deprive your body of important nutrients you need to perform at your best.

3. FUEL WITH MINIMALLY PROCESSED CARBOHYDRATES

Background: Carbohydrates have gotten a bad rap for more than a decade and will continue to be a polarizing topic. There should be no debate that active people who want to boost mental focus and physical performance need to meet those energy needs with the right carbohydrates.

Carbs are our primary fuel source. They provide energy for muscle function and act as the main fuel for the brain. When you don't take in enough carbs, your body does not run efficiently or effectively. Think of carbs as the fuel for your body's gas tank. If you don't eat enough carbs, you'll run out of fuel, which means low energy, decreased focus, and even nasty mood swings.

When carbs are broken down, glucose (the primary fuel for the brain and body) is made available. The more processed the carbohydrate, the faster that happens and the less stable the energy it provides. A less-processed food will provide more stable energy and less of a glucose and insulin spike. Uncontrolled blood sugar has been linked to an increased risk of inflammation, cardiovascular disease, diabetes, and a negative impact on the brain.

Make It Happen: Not all carbs are created equal. Avoid processed carbs such as white breads, pastas, and baked goods. These have a high glycemic index, meaning they're digested quickly and absorbed immediately, sending your blood sugar level sky-high. The problem is, you crash quickly and end up feeling sluggish.

Instead, choose the least-processed carbs available. Low- or moderate-glycemic foods cause the body to do the work to extract the nutrients in the foods, and that gradual release helps regulate blood sugar. Think "Brown and Close to the Ground," a reference to both the color of the carbs and where the food was grown. Choose carbohydrates and grains with at least 3 grams of fiber to stabilize energy, keep you feeling full, and protect your heart. Great choices include steel-cut oats, quinoa, kamut, lentils, 100 percent whole wheat bread, and sweet potatoes.

Include fruits, vegetables, beans, and whole grains for their fiber and nutrient density.

Your meals should revolve around nutrient-dense colorful foods, and that includes carbs, too. Choose the least-processed form. If you opt for pasta or couscous, select the whole wheat option. If you reach for rice, opt for brown rice or wild rice.

4. POWER WITH LEAN PROTEINS

Background: Lean protein plays a key role in stabilizing our energy levels, providing nutrients to our body for recovery and repair, and protecting our immune function. Research shows that those who get the protein they need throughout the day maintain muscle mass and are leaner than those that don't. Athletes don't need more than 1 gram of protein per pound of body weight per day.

That might sound like a lot of protein—and it is a significant amount—but consider how much protein is in these common foods:

Chicken (4 ounces, skinless, the size of a deck of cards): 35 grams

Cod or salmon (6 ounces): 40 grams

Tuna (6 ounces, packed in water): 40 grams

Lean pork (4 ounces): 35 grams

Lean red meat (4 ounces): 35 grams

Tofu (6 ounces): 30 grams

Cottage cheese (1 cup, 1% or 2% fat): 28 grams

Milk (1 cup or 1%, 2% or fat-free): 8 grams

1 egg: 6 grams

1 egg white: 3 grams

Make It Happen: Protein intake should be split up over the course of the day, and it should be included in every meal or snack to meet your needs of 0.8 to 1 gram per pound per day. If you weigh 180 pounds, for instance, you would need roughly 180 grams of protein per day. Dividing that by six meals comes to 30 grams of protein per feeding. Protein helps to stabilize energy, promotes satiety, and also revs up the metabolism. Your body has to work a little harder to digest protein; therefore your metabolism gets a bit of a jolt each time you include it in a meal. By including a protein source with each of your meals and your postworkout recovery shake, you will easily and effectively satisfy your protein needs.

Great protein choices are fish, chicken, eggs, low-fat dairy, Greek yogurt, beans, and legumes.

When it comes to selecting protein, remember this rule: The Less Legs, the Better. The fewer legs on the animal the protein came from, the better it is for you. Fish don't have legs, of course. Always choose grilled instead of fried, white meat instead of dark, and skinless instead of with skin.

You also should incorporate a postworkout recovery shake into your routine. That mix will contain 10 to 25 grams of protein per serving, along with carbs. If you have one or two shakes a day, along with some combination of poultry and fish for lunch and dinner and a breakfast that includes yogurt or eggs, you'll easily meet your daily protein goal.

5. EAT FATS THAT GIVE BACK

Background: The right types of fats are powerful protectors of the body. Fats are crucial to good health and the makeup of cell membranes. Fats are needed for the absorption of certain vitamins and antioxidants. They release energy slowly, keeping the body satiated and regulating blood sugar, thus lowering glycemic response to other foods. Good fats provide powerful nutrients for cellular repair of the joints, organs, skin, and hair. Omega-3 fatty acids improve cognition, decrease inflammation, and enhance heart health. Omega-3 fatty acids are considered essential because your body cannot make them; you must get them through food. People typically do not get nearly enough omega-3 fatty acids in their diets, resulting in subpar brain function and increased inflammation in the body. Healthy fats are found in fatty fish like salmon, trout, and tuna, as well as flaxseed, hemp, walnuts, and omega-3 fortified foods.

Make It Happen: Ensure that you include healthy fats at each meal with an enhanced focus on omega-3 fatty acids. Great fat sources are found in nuts (pecans, almonds, walnuts), natural nut butters, olive oil, and avocado. Foods rich in omega-3 fatty acids are walnuts, salmon, tuna, fish oil, flaxseed and flaxseed oil, hemp, and chia seeds.

6. EAT THE RAINBOW

Background: When you look at your plate, you should see a rainbow—a lot of color in the form of fruits, vegetables, and high-fiber grains. Our bodies need vitamins, minerals, antioxidants, and enzymes to perform. Fruits and vegetables provide nutrients the way nature designed. Both fruits and veggies provide our bodies with nutrients, but we need to focus on a variety of color coming from a number of sources. Fruits tend to be consumed more often, and we need to focus on our deep green leafy veggies and ensure those are incorporated on a regular basis.

Make It Happen: You cannot go wrong with any fruit or vegetable; however, these pack a serious punch: deep green leafy vegetables (kale, spinach, Swiss chard), berries, peppers, and beets.

3 | EAT OFTEN

Long gone is that 1970s philosophy of eating three square meals a day and avoiding between-meal snacks. Today, we know that if you want to control your blood sugar level and energy level to improve concentration, regulate your appetite, and build lean body mass, you must eat six small- to medium-size meals or snacks a day. That means you need to eat, on average, every three hours. Think of yourself as fueling throughout the day instead of sitting for three big meals. If you can't control your blood sugar levels, you're going to have wild fluctuations in energy levels and moods and an impaired ability to concentrate.

Like a fire, your metabolism is in constant need of fuel. If you let it go for a long time without adding logs, the fire smolders and dies. Each time you eat (or add fuel to the fire), it cranks up your metabolism and burns more calories to digest the food. You have an efficient metabolism.

By following the Athletes' Performance program, you'll create this constantly burning fire. If you don't continually fuel the fire, you're going to draw from your valuable lean muscle mass and smolder. If you don't eat often, the most readily available substance for the body to consume is muscle—not fat, as is commonly believed.

7. EAT BREAKFAST EVERY DAY

Background: Breakfast is, indeed, the most important meal of the day. Your body has been fasting since you went to bed, so it's important that you "break the fast" not long after rising and keep your body fueled all day long. When you eat within thirty minutes of waking up, you jump-start your metabolism and fuel your brain. This gives you more energy to get your day going.

Make It Happen: Breakfast should include protein, carbs, fruits and vegetables, and fit fats. Examples include whole grain toast with natural peanut butter, yogurt, and a banana; oatmeal, berries, almonds, and a hard-boiled egg; and an English muffin with scrambled eggs and avocado with 100 percent fruit juice.

8. EAT EVERY THREE HOURS

Background: Eating small meals more often controls appetite and regulates blood sugar, promotes muscle mass, improves concentration, and eliminates mood swings and overeating.

Make It Happen: After breakfast, eat smaller meals more often, spread evenly across the day. No excuses; you should be eating four to six meals per day. Aim for all three macronutrients (carbs, proteins, and fat) every three hours for proper fueling.

4 | HYDRATE

For all of the advances in technology, we still have not come up with something better to drink than water. Unfortunately, though, we tend to replace it with inferior beverages, ranging from soda to coffee to alcohol. Or we simply don't drink enough. Drinking can be a bit of an afterthought, with food and fueling taking front and center, but hydration should be something that we are proactive with—and give equal attention.

Drinking sufficient water increases energy, improves the quality of skin and fascia, keeps muscles and joints lubricated, improves overall health, and prevents overeating. Hydration impacts your brain and your mental ability. Water is available for little to no cost, and you can drink as much as you'd like.

Dehydration translates into decreased performance. A deficit of just half a liter of water can cause an increase in the stress hormone cortisol, and even slight dehydration can negatively affect mood.

By drinking the proper amount of water every day, you could accomplish 25 percent more. Proper hydration regulates appetite. Often when people think they're hungry, they're really just thirsty. Staying hydrated throughout the day will help you achieve your ideal body composition. Get in touch with your hunger by asking yourself if you are truly hungry or just thirsty.

Water can retard the aging process. Because of dehydration, inactivity, and trauma from daily life, the fascia and connective tissues around our muscles and joints dry up over time. Meeting your hydration needs prevents this process while improving your muscle tissue and flexibility.

When you think about it, there's no excuse not to stay hydrated.

9. MEET YOUR FOUNDATIONAL HYDRATION NEEDS

Background: The Institute of Medicine (IOM) recommends that men consume 3.7 liters and women consume 2.7 liters of fluid per day. This fluid should be calorie free. Sports drinks are designed for intense sport, not for supporting foundational hydration.

Don't drink calories. It's the single easiest way to get a handle on your nutrition program. If you replace soft drinks, juices, sports drinks, and alcohol with water or natural teas, you'll cut down on calories and sugar.

Make It Happen: Drink ½ to 1 ounce of fluid per pound per day. This should be made up of water and other naturally calorie-free beverages, like green tea. Jump-start your hydration by beginning your day with 16 ounces of water as soon as you wake up.

> **Remember:** The most effective way to maintain performance is to start your Performance Day hydrated. The only way to do this is to meet your hydration needs throughout the day—every day.

Body Weight (lbs)	Ounces of Fluid Per Day	Liters Per Day
120	60–120	2–4
150	75–150	2.5–5
175	90–175	3–6
200	100–200	3.5–7
225	115–200	4–8
250	125–200	4.5–9

If you're unsure of your hydration level, take a look at your urine. If it's a clear or pale lemonade color, you're hydrated. If it's a darker lemonade to apple juice color, you're dehydrated. And if it's dark and cloudy, you're severely dehydrated and should seek medical attention.

10. STAY HYDRATED DURING ACTIVITY

Background: Losing just 2 percent of your body weight due to fluid loss decreases performance. If you are a heavy "salty" sweater or are training in an extreme environment, it is important to pay attention to the sodium content of your beverage. Cramping has been linked to electrolyte loss, specifically sodium loss. Choose a hydration beverage that has at least 200 milligrams of sodium per 8 ounces to maximize electrolyte replacement.

The amount of fluid lost (measured as a loss of body weight over the course of your session) is an indicator as to your risk of a decrease in performance and eventually heat illness. The more weight you lose, the more serious the impact to performance and health.

Make It Happen:

- Pretraining (1–2 hours before), drink 17–20 ounces.
- Immediately before training, drink 7–10 ounces.
- During training (every 10–15 minutes), drink 7–10 ounces.
- Post-training, drink 20 ounces for every pound lost.

How Alcohol Negatively Affects Performance

Alcohol is not part of a high-performance lifestyle. I'm not going to tell you to abstain. Just recognize that alcohol decreases performance potential by up to 11.4 percent. It increases the release of the stress hormone cortisol, impacts the immune system, and decreases protein synthesis for muscle fiber repair. Alcohol diminishes water-soluble vitamins required for hormones to do their work, impairs reaction time up to twelve hours after consumption, disturbs REM sleep, and decreases the body's ability to recover.

If you're going to drink, limit yourself to one or two drinks per week. If you're going to have more than that, then I hope you'll have drinks with some health benefit, such as red wines, which have flavonoids that act as antioxidants. (If you drink beer, be sure to factor the carbs into your daily intake.) Always drink one glass of water for every alcoholic drink, as alcohol is a diuretic.

Bottom line: If you want to be dialed in to piss excellence and be a high performer, alcohol is not part of the game plan.

5 | RECOVER

By now you should be thinking of nutrition in terms of *fueling* your body. But it's also a key part of recovery.

Most people think of eating and recovering in terms of Thanksgiving dinner or other big meals. A "food coma" sets in that leaves you lethargic and wanting to fall asleep in front of the television.

Rather than recovering *from* eating, we want to think in terms of fueling *to* recover. This pertains not only to our postworkout recovery fueling (more on that in a moment), but also how we use food to kick-start our day-to-day recovery from the stresses of life.

11. FUEL FOR YOUR ACTIVITY

Background: You never want to be deprived of key nutrients, especially when you train. Yet many people train first thing in the morning on an empty stomach. Training, of course, is a great way to start the day. But eat something before you train, even if it's just half an apple with a handful of nuts, a slice of whole wheat toast with natural peanut butter, yogurt, or a preworkout shooter consisting of a half glass of watered-down orange juice with a scoop of whey protein. To maximize your performance on the field or training floor, you need to start off fueled. Your focus should be on carbohydrate (Fuel) with a little bit of protein (Build).

Make It Happen: Regardless of what time of day you train, it's crucial to fuel properly beforehand. Great preworkout fuel includes: yogurt with ½ cup of berries and ¾ cup of high-fiber cereal; a small bowl of cereal with a banana; half a turkey sandwich and fruit; half a peanut butter and jelly sandwich and fruit; or homemade trail mix consisting of 1 cup of high-fiber cereal, 2 tablespoons of dried fruit, and 2 tablespoons of nuts. Be sure to hydrate with 16 to 20 ounces of water.

12. STAY FUELED DURING YOUR ACTIVITY

Background: You never want to run out of fuel during training. Endurance athletes know this as bonking, where they are forced to slow down or even stop due to insufficient nutrition or hydration. Regardless of your training, you'll experience a similar deficit and frustration if you don't take the proper nutritional measures. You want to maintain your fuel stores during training so that you can perform at a higher level throughout the session, but also to maintain energy reserves for a strong finish.

Make It Happen: Regardless of the intensity of your training session, consume 7 to 10 ounces of fluid (about 4 to 6 gulps) every fifteen minutes. If the session is more than forty-five minutes long or is in intense heat, choose a sports drink with at least 200 milligrams of sodium per 8 ounces to help prevent cramping and maintain electrolytes. When your training level warrants the consumption of a sports drink for performance benefits, you'll want to consume the equivalent of 30 to 60 grams of carbs per hour. This will ensure that you are properly fueled and feeling great during the session. All you need to stay fueled is 20 to 32 ounces an hour. Balance the rest of your hydration needs with water.

13. REFUEL AND REBUILD AFTER YOUR WORKOUT

Background: After a workout, the body is in a breakdown (catabolic) state. We want to be in a building (anabolic) state. Recovery fueling increases blood insulin levels, lowers blood cortisol levels, strengthens the immune system, restores muscle and livery glycogen, and stimulates muscle protein synthesis and repair.

One of our top goals is to create more intelligent lean mass. That in turn will burn more calories, both at rest and during training. If we don't eat immediately following a workout, our bodies will first turn to our hard-earned lean mass for energy. As much as we'd like to think it would turn to our fat stores, the body doesn't work that way. By losing lean mass, you're creating a body that burns calories *less* efficiently.

Make It Happen: When you've finished a workout, your cells are wide open and screaming for nutrients. The quickest and easiest way to replenish them is to consume, within ten minutes of training, a postworkout recovery shake made with a protein powder (or supplement), such as 100 percent whey protein blended with a

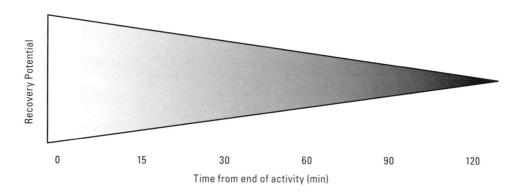

banana or EAS Recovery Protein. Prepackaged shake mixes contain an effective ratio of proteins, carbohydrates, and fat and are loaded with fiber, vitamins, and minerals. Since the shakes can be made by mixing water with a scoop or packet of powder in a covered plastic container or blender, they make a quick, easy, and portable meal that won't spoil.

By having a shake right after your workout, you expedite the recovery process and maximize lean muscle growth. Protein powder shakes that combine the right ratio of carbohydrate and protein have been a longtime component of our Athletes' Performance training centers, and the elite-level athletes who train with us have long benefited from these products. If you go through the effort to train and move your body and don't take measures to repair it, you've wasted your workout. In fact, you've done damage to your body by breaking it down without taking measures to repair it.

Whichever product you choose, look for something that's going to provide the right mix of protein and carbs (see chart below).

Compared with your training session, postworkout nutrition is the easy part. We train to get stronger, fitter, more powerful, and more efficient, but without postworkout nutrition you will be missing an opportunity to maximize your adaptations to training and may never achieve your full potential. If you don't want to consume a shake, that's fine. Depending on when you work out, just move your regularly scheduled meal or fueling to within thirty minutes of your workout. Just make sure you get something with a combination of carbohydrates and protein in your system within thirty minutes of training (ideally ten). It will improve your energy, speed your recovery, and keep you feeling great while training day in and day out.

What do you need to recover?

Body Weight (lbs)	Grams of Protein	Grams of Carbs
120–149	20–25	50–60
150–180	25–30	60–75
181–215	30–35	75–90
215–245	35–40	90–105

14. FOUNDATIONAL NUTRITION SUPPORT

Background: By following the Athletes' Performance nutritional program, you will fuel your body for high performance. The foundational nutrition strategies

Traveling Nutritional Strategies

You have less control over what and when you eat when you're traveling. If you want to make smart nutritional choices when you're on the road, don't leave the house empty-handed. Stay hydrated. Drink ½ to 1 ounce of water per pound of body weight every day. This is especially important with air travel. Aim to drink about 8 ounces of fluid every hour on the plane.

Your Travel Checklist—Don't Travel Without It!
Shaker bottle (for shakes)
Water container or bottled water
Green tea bags
High-fiber cereal, granola bars, EAS bars, or bars of choice
EAS shake packets, shake packet of choice, or 100 percent whey protein in a
    Ziploc bag
Nuts, seeds, dried fruit, and high-fiber cereal mix
Individual servings of natural peanut butter
Instant oatmeal
Fresh fruit and veggies (apple, banana, orange, carrots)
Beef jerky, hard-boiled eggs, or low-fat cheese
Sandwiches (pita, tortillas, bread)
Whole grain crackers (must have at least 3 grams of fiber)
(Note: Ziploc bags and plastic utensils should always be in stock in your
    kitchen.)

The single most important step in eating well when traveling is to take control of your food choices. When choosing food at airports, look for a sandwich shop and take something onto the plane. Keep your food and water accessible when you are on the plane.

Breakfast choices: eggs, oatmeal, high-fiber cereal, yogurt, peanut butter, fruit
Lunch/dinner choices: lean meat, whole grain bread, whole wheat pasta,
    regular pasta, brown rice, fruit and veggies
Between-meal fuel: meal replacement bars, shakes, sandwich, fruit, veggies,
    nuts, beef jerky

Smart Travel Reminders

1. Don't skip meals: You must eat every three hours.
2. Bring bars and shakes: These are great for light fueling and pre-/postworkout nutrition.
3. Make sure there is a lean protein choice with each meal: Grilled chicken, filet of beef, grilled fish, grilled pork, turkey, ham, and roast beef are great on sandwiches. Avoid anything fried.
4. Add your grains, wholesome carbs, fruits, and veggies: Add baked potato, rice, pasta, whole wheat bread, fresh fruit or veggies to every meal.
5. Stay hydrated! Drink ½ to 1 ounce per pound of body weight per day. This is especially important with air travel. Aim to drink about 8 ounces of fluid every hour on the plane.
6. Hunt at the airport: Amidst all of the restaurants at the airport, search out the sandwich shops and the kiosks. You can build a great sandwich or salad and find trail mix, nuts, bars, and water at any kiosk or airport store.
7. Write it down: If you have problems keeping your travel nutrition in check, take a small notebook with you when you travel and journal what you eat and drink during the trip.

provided in this section will give you everything you need to thrive throughout your Performance Day. Vitamins are catalysts that regulate reactions in your body. You must get vitamins from your diet because your body cannot make them. Nutritional deficiencies develop over the course of months or years of inadequate intake. There is no pill that can completely replicate the delicate balance of vitamins, minerals, and phytochemicals that occur naturally in food. But there is no denying that you need vitamins for your body to function at a high level; therefore, if you are not getting everything you need from food, supplements can be a part of your Performance Day.

Make It Happen: A multivitamin that offers a full spectrum of antioxidants and B vitamins can fill in the gaps of your nutrition plan, sending in reinforcements in the fight against cellular-damaging free radicals, keeping our bodies and minds healthy. Fish oil provides powerful omega-3 fatty acids, which have anti-inflammatory properties and are essential for good cardiovascular health and mental clarity. The omega-3 fatty acids found in wild salmon, mackerel, lake trout, herring, sardines, tuna, and some types of whitefish cannot be made by your body, so they must come from your diet. Unless you eat fish at least three times a week, you're not getting enough omega-3s. Everyone should have a bottle of fish oil or fish oil capsules in the pantry. If fish oil gives you a case of the burps, krill oil is a good substitute.

Vitamin D, also known as the sunlight vitamin, is an essential vitamin that helps increase immunity, improve bone health, reduce stress, and regulate blood pressure. Your body can make vitamin D by absorbing UVB rays from the sun through your skin.

If you live in an area with little sun exposure, wear a lot of sunscreen, or follow a vegan diet, you might not be getting enough vitamin D. An additional 600 IUs a day will help ensure you have adequate daily vitamin D. Before starting any new complement (aka supplement), make sure you talk with your doctor or medical professional. Whenever possible, it is best to have your blood work done prior to picking your supplement doses.

Supplement Safety

The supplement industry is crowded with companies that sell products that are unethical and unsafe, and may never have been tested against their claims. What is in the product is not guaranteed to be on the label, and what is on the label is not guaranteed to be in the product, unless the supplement has gone through third-party testing. For the professional athlete, this can mean testing positive for a banned substance. For the military operator, this can mean taking a supplement that may have a negative impact on your health without knowing it. For the performance-minded individual, this can mean wasting your hard-earned money on a product that will never live up to its claims. Your best bet to confirm the safety and efficacy of a product is to ensure that the product has gone through third-party testing. The two testing bodies out there that we trust most are NSF (www.nsfsport.com) and Informed-Choice (www.informed-choice.org).

15. COMPLEMENT YOUR TRAINING

Background: At EXOS, we prefer to think not in terms of supplements, but rather in terms of nutritional options that *complement* our training and foundational nutrition.

Food is always the first priority, followed by these complementary options that will take your performance to another level in a safe and ethical way. At Athletes' Performance, we're advocates of EAS products, not only because EAS is a long-time partner of ours, but also because EAS was the first to obtain NSF (National Sanitation Foundation) certification, which guarantees that products are banned-substance-free and meet high standards for labeling accuracy.

Here are some complementary options to consider:

HMB: Muscles are damaged during training, causing muscle protein to break down. HMB (hydroxy methylbutyrate), a metabolite of leucine (a branched-chain amino acid), helps prevent protein breakdown. The amount of HMB needed to produce the benefits of muscle development is 3 grams each day. Your body produces some HMB naturally from the amino acid leucine, but only small amounts of leucine are converted to HMB. Thus, it is easier and more efficient to supplement directly with HMB as opposed to leucine to get the desired daily amount of HMB. Taking HMB daily is recommended so that it's always in your bloodstream, constantly helping you achieve a strong, lean body composition.

BETA ALANINE: A naturally occurring amino acid, beta alanine makes a compound in your body called carnosine, which controls the buildup of hydrogen ions in your muscles caused by intense or prolonged exercise. The buildup of hydrogen is a major factor in causing muscles to fatigue, using beta alanine can help delay it. This allows you to build more muscle, increase your strength, and improve your explosive power.

The amount of beta alanine needed to get the benefit of delayed muscle fatigue and more intense training is between 3 and 6.4 grams per day in divided doses. You get some beta alanine in your daily diet, but typically only 15 to 20 percent of what your muscles need to control acid accumulation. We recommend consuming beta alanine in divided doses throughout the day. You can split up your doses around your training with the first coming sixty to ninety minutes before training and the second within two hours of finishing.

CREATINE: Contrary to popular belief, creatine is not magic pixie dust to make you huge. It is one of the most well-researched ergogenic aids on the market.

In the 1990s, it was linked to muscle pulls and kidney damage, but those concerns have long been debunked. If your foundational nutrition is sound, creatine can be effective in helping you fuel muscles and recover from repeated short bursts of explosive movement.

Creatine is naturally found in animal products, especially meat. One pound of raw meat, however, contains only 1 to 2 grams of creatine. Your body synthesizes 1 to 2 grams of creatine a day, primarily in the liver, kidneys, and pancreas.

Creatine has been found to increase strength and maximal power by up to 15 percent, and can also improve lean body mass. Optimal levels of creatine can enhance your muscles' ability to renew energy for up to twenty-second energy bursts.

Creatine can support brain function, especially if you are vegetarian, vegan, or low in creatine. A study showed that vegetarians who took 5 grams of creatine per day for six weeks had better working memory and speed of processing.

To increase your body's stores of creatine, take 5 grams daily. Some advocate a load phase of 20 grams a day for seven days, but at Athletes' Performance we recommend 5 grams per day, which is sufficient.

CAFFEINE: If you're getting adequate sleep and following the Athletes' Performance nutrition program, you should not need caffeine just to get through the day. But when used on occasion, it's a proven training aid for athletes. Caffeine stimulates the central nervous system, causes the body to use fat as fuel more ef-

Remember: Check Off Your Daily Nutritional Strategies for Your Performance Day

View food as fuel

Hit 80/20

Fuel with minimally processed
   carbohydrates

Power with lean proteins

Eat fats that give back

Eat the rainbow

Eat breakfast every day

Eat every three hours

Meet your foundational hydration needs

Stay hydrated during activity

Fuel for your activity

Stay fueled during your activity

Refuel and rebuild after your workout

Foundational nutrition support

Complement your training

fectively, and preserves muscle glycogen. You'll feel more energetic, and your perceived rate of exertion will be lower.

Our research at Athletes' Performance has found that caffeine significantly improves peak power outputs, especially when athletes need a special push. A dose of 75 to 200 milligrams has been shown to give you a meaningful boost. Check with your doctor before using caffeine if you have high blood pressure or a heart condition.

Again, caffeine is not something you want to use on a regular basis. You'll develop a tolerance for it and minimize its effectiveness. That could inspire you to take heavier doses, leading to dependency and other system complications. But when used sparingly, it can be a valuable boost to performance.

Simple Guide to Supplements

Nutrient	Performance Support	Dosing
HMB	Improved efficiency in muscle protein protection	1.5 g twice per day
Beta Alanine	Improves buffering capability during high intensity exercise, resulting in increased ability to maintain performance at high workloads	1.5 to 3.2 g twice per day
Creatine	Improves ability to perform during repeated high intensity and explosive movements	5 g per day if less than 290 lb body weight, 10 g per day if greater than 290 lb body weight
Caffeine	Central nervous system stimulation Delays fatigue	1 to 3 mg per kg body mass 45 minutes pre-exercise
Probiotics	Provides healthy bacteria to protect the gut and maximize immune function	10 to 50 billion CFU (colony forming units) per day
Whey Protein or Protein Blends	Provides amino acids for muscle recovery	0.3 to 0.4 g per kg of lean body mass post workout
Multivitamin	Fills in the requirements around a lacking diet	1 per day (or as recommended)
Fish Oil	Anti-inflammatory properties Supports cardiovascular health Supports mental clarity	1 to 3 g EPA/DHA per day

Athletes' Performance Power Foods

We've already discussed plenty of nutritious foods from which you can build tasty, nutrient-dense meals. But there are some foods that are especially valuable when it comes to fueling your Performance Day. These nutrient-rich options are packed with vitamins, antioxidants, and fiber, providing a powerful punch in usually a small amount of calories.

Some of these foods no doubt will be familiar to you, but perhaps you've never considered how valuable they are in terms of fueling your success. Some you might have dismissed after one tasting in childhood. You know what? It's time to give them another chance. High performers recognize that there always are new (or old) methods to take their games to another level, and nutrition is no exception.

Some of these foods, in addition to being highly nutritious, provide taste and texture to meals, which is always important. When it comes to nutrition, it's hard to beat foods that are both tasty and good for you.

That's why we call these fifty foods our Athletes' Performance Power Foods.

Almonds	Coconut	Kale	Rosemary
Artichokes	Collard greens	Kefir	Salmon
Avocados	Dark chocolate	Kiwi	Sardines
Beans	Edamame	Lentils	Spinach
Beets	Eggs	Olive oil	Steel-cut oats
Berries	Farro	Oregano	Sunflower seeds
Broccoli	Flaxseeds	Oysters	Sweet potatoes/
Brussels sprouts	Garlic	Parsley	yams
Buffalo	Ginger	Pecans	Swiss chard
Cherries	Grass-fed beef	Pistachios	Thyme
Chia seeds	Greek yogurt	Pomegranates	Turmeric
Cinnamon	Green tea	Pumpkin	Walnuts
Citrus fruits	Hemp seeds	Quinoa	

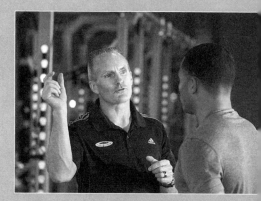

3 | TRAIN FOR IT

Athletes' Performance Movement

TO BE YOUR BEST, YOU NEED TO UNDERSTAND THE SCIENCE OF MOVEMENT
Regardless of your sport or whether you're a tactical athlete, movement is the common thread among all athletes.

You might think you move well now, but at EXOS we've never seen an athlete that has not improved speed, power, and endurance by improving the efficiency of movement patterns. Moving efficiently improves performance and keeps you from suffering injuries.

We view the body and how it moves as an integrated system. We don't draw walls between various body groups, systems, and body parts; it's one system.

When we introduced the Core Performance system through our first book more than a decade ago, it represented a paradigm shift for the industry to train movement patterns to improve on-field performance. We all grew up following some training category: power lifting, Olympic lifting, bodybuilding, or endurance training. Those were the choices, but, as with everything else, you can find more effective ways to do something.

Our responsibility to our clients is to show them how to improve their on-field performance, whether that's the field of sport or the field of battle. That's the essence of this book: to teach you that system.

These days, in the YouTube world of online experts, there exist countless exercises that you *could* do or that perhaps would be nice to do. You can train someone in any number of ways, but there are only a few proven methods that show how to move efficiently, perform at a high level, and reduce the risk of injury.

It is frustrating to see professionals in our field asking people to tackle challenges and enter situations when they're unprepared. These "experts" are putting people in harm's way, resulting in injury and failure, which is unnecessary with the level of knowledge and research that exists today. We recognize that you're highly valued by your organization, to say nothing of your family, and in most cases irreplaceable. Keeping you injury-free and performing at the highest level is our top priority.

We want to make you aware of how your body is supposed to move, which you've probably lost track of over the years. The body is a phenomenal compensator, and you've likely adapted to it moving, like a car out of alignment, at a level that's adequate but far from ideal.

Unfortunately we don't have the luxury of evaluating you personally. So we looked at the various populations that we see in the sport and tactical athlete space. Based on the average of their evaluative data, we engineered the solution to address the majority of what we see to decrease the potential for injury and improve performance.

As with any high-performance vehicle, your movement, like the chassis of a car, needs to be maintained and serviced so it can provide the foundation to your technical skills, whether we're talking a specific sport or a military endeavor.

We stress the power and efficiency of effective movement patterns. These are the prerequisites to high performance. Yet the vast majority of elite athletes we see have major deficiencies in these fundamental movement patterns. They possess the equivalent of software viruses obtained from overly aggressive or incorrect training methods. It's also a product of poor habits and posture, along with not recovering from hard training. Perhaps you've been a high performer to this point, but you've paid a price to get here.

When athletes arrive at one of our training centers, we use one of more than a dozen movement screens to evaluate them. It's no different from the diagnostic checkup a mechanic performs on a car. These screens typically reveal a lack of stability and poor mobility (range of motion).

In this program, we give you the tools to constantly evaluate yourself, to be your own movement screen. The program itself will be a constant evaluation tool as you recognize and attack any imbalances in your body. You'll need to take note either by how it feels, how it looks in the mirror, how much weight you use, or how easily you can perform a movement. Is one side easier than the other? If so, that's a red flag to focus upon. More than 70 percent of injuries in elite sport and the military are not from trauma, but rather from these imbalances that over time produce injuries. It's not a matter of *if* it will happen, but *when*. This is what sidelines athletes from being able to train and compete at the highest level and what cuts careers short. You might not think it's a big deal when you're young. After all, it's like you're a new car. But it becomes more challenging with each ten thousand miles you log on your body, which is the vehicle to your success.

In a recent study undertaken by Arizona State University and the University of South Florida, sixty-one individuals were identified to have risk for injury using the Functional Movement Screen, one of the most respected screens in the field, developed by Gray Cook. The group was placed on the Athletes' Performance training systems for three days a week. After three weeks, 69 percent no longer were at risk of injury. After six weeks, 90 percent no longer were at risk.

So take note of these imbalances and use the tools in this book to correct them. Practice these moves until they become second nature, giving you the confidence that comes from having the power to master this system.

This awareness might come during the Foundation Phase in the form of an inability to execute a movement or get your body in the proper position. This is going to be uncomfortable and frustrating. You might view this as not worth the trouble and perhaps endure ridicule from colleagues who stay in that same stubborn mindset. Let them remain in the same place they've been for the last five to ten years while you are launching to a new level.

The reason you will continue to achieve is that you're able to learn new skills, moving forward with an open mind to perfect anything you focus upon. This is what defines a high performer. If you continue to do the things you like and are good at, you will be one-dimensional and not grow. This is about improving your performance.

In this training program, we are going to talk a lot about power principles. We're going to share many ways to improve mobility, stability, and movement pattern efficiency while increasing strength, power, and endurance.

The goal is to clean up the movements needed to perform your tasks better. This program will improve the efficiency of your movement, decreasing the stress and load on your body and allowing you to recover more quickly.

Regardless of your training environment, which could range from world-class facilities and staff to a bare-bones gym membership, you will be able to apply the majority of these movements and concepts and still get the results you would in an ideal environment. There are no excuses in this book, just results. We want to put you in a situation to achieve results any time, any place, because you understand the principles of the Athletes' Performance Training System and are empowered to act upon them.

ATHLETES' PERFORMANCE MOVEMENT

1. Pillar Prep
2. Movement Prep
3. Plyometrics
4. Movement Skills
5. Medicine Ball
6. Relative Power
7. Energy Systems Development (ESD)

1 | Pillar Prep

The title of this section is "Pillar Prep," but that just refers to the movements at the beginning of our training session. Pillar strength is a concept that encompasses training movements that involve the shoulders, torso (or core), and hips. All movement involves the pillar, as energy is both generated from it and transferred through it. If the pillar lacks stability and/or mobility, the result is inefficient movement and energy leaks. These inefficient movement patterns and energy leaks lead to decreased performance and a greater risk of injury.

The pillar gives us a center axis from which to move. Traditional workout programs think of warm-ups in terms of activating the legs and arms. It makes sense instead to first warm up the pillar. That's the role of Pillar Prep; it's a brief series of movements that activates and strengthens the pillar, providing great stability before progressing to more challenging movements.

In order to have the best pillar strength, we need to have perfect posture and be as symmetrical as possible. Contrary to popular belief, no athlete is ever perfectly symmetrical. Even at birth, the body is not perfectly symmetrical, but the body as a whole is a perfectly balanced system.

Living in a sedentary culture and training improperly locks down our hips and creates asymmetry in our bodies, which leads to dysfunction and injury. We want to get back to the same near-perfect movement patterns we had as babies. When we can build that pillar strength, we're able to move more efficiently and with more force.

Pillar strength is important because each movement requires stretching muscles, and one end is usually attached within your pillar region. Through this stable pillar, we're able to capture energy and transfer force, making the body more elastic and efficient at producing speed, power, and endurance with less effort.

Sounds good, right? Unfortunately, after the rigors athletes go through for the demands of their game and preparation, their pillars look like the equivalent of a twelve-year-old car that's been driven into the ground. Our athletes arrive with some hard miles on their odometers. Chances are you're in the same position.

We typically see athletes with their shoulders and necks rolled inward and protruding forward. This is caused by having a tight upper body (pectorals, lats, and trapezii), which creates what's known as upper cross syndrome, that hunched-forward look that robs an athlete of power and even affects breathing.

The good news is that we can roll back your odometer, strengthening your pillar to rediscover your proper alignment and power potential. If you think of how a child learns to move, beginning with a forearm commando crawl and progressing to crawling on the hands and finally to pulling themselves upright, it's a similar process that you will undertake to rekindle these movements and produce pillar strength.

Pillar strength is the integration of the shoulder, torso, and hips across the three planes of motion: frontal, sagittal, and transverse.

The frontal plane bisects the body to create front and back halves, creating an anterior-posterior axis. Frontal plane movements include lateral pillar bridges, cutting while keeping your body inside your base of support, or lateral lunges.

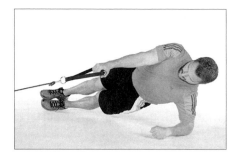

The sagittal plane bisects the body to create left and right sides, creating motion around a coronal axis. Sagittal plane movements include flexion and extension movements such as squatting, deadlifts, and marching.

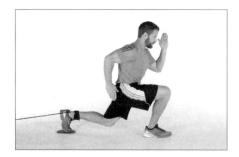

The transverse plane bisects the body to create upper and lower halves, creating a longitudinal or vertical axis. Transverse plane movements include internal and external rotation of the limbs, rotational medicine ball throwing, and swinging a bat or golf club.

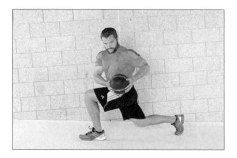

Hip Stability: The hip cuff is the lower body's control unit. It governs the thigh, which interacts with your knee and affects your foot position. The central location of the hip cuff is why care must be paid to strengthening the muscles in and around the area, as they are critical in controlling everything below your hips and everything above as well.

The hip cuff consists of more than forty muscles in and around your pelvis, 40 percent of which cause internal or external rotation of the hip, which are responsible for much of your lower body movement and power. Hips are the most overlooked area when it comes to decreasing the potential for injury and improving performance. Most back and hip problems occur because of improper mobility and stability and improper use of the hips. Most people are locked down or unstable in their hips. If one of your hip capsules is locked down, it's as if one of your thighbones is welded to your pelvis—imagine wearing a permanent cast on your hip.

This program, starting with Pillar Prep, will help you develop more femoral control by focusing not on your knees but on the hip cuff. We'll spend lots of time on movements that challenge the hip cuff.

Torso (Core) Stability: Torso stability is much more than a chiseled midsection or washboard abs. The core consists of the muscles of your torso. It's the vital link between hip and shoulder stability, and it includes the bone, joint, and muscle groups such as the rectus abdominis, transverse abdominis, internal and external obliques, pelvic floor, psoas, diaphragm, erector spinae, latissimi dorsi (lats), and many small stabilizing muscles between the vertebrae of the spine, known as the multifidi.

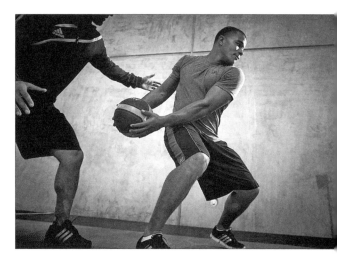

The multifidi are the tiny muscles that often get shut off because of a back injury and never become reactivated, causing long-term back problems. These muscles cannot function alone; you have to help them by training your core muscles to become strong and stable, with the right types of recruitment patterns that will enable them to work in tandem with your shoulders and hips.

In order to get the benefit of the movements in this program, you must keep your torso active and aligned, not just while training, but all day. Think of your stomach flat against the hip bones. Keep your stomach tight, as if pulling off your belt buckle. This isn't the same as sucking in your gut and holding your breath. Keep the abdominals in, but still breathe.

Mastering your breathing patterns (more on that later) and Pillar Preparation will ensure your torso is supported from the outside in and the inside out, so you'll be well on your way to efficient movement and preventing long-term deterioration. With this program, it will work into your subconscious and become automatic.

Shoulder Stability: We tend to think of the hands and arms as carrying the workload for the upper body, but it's really the shoulders that should bear or "shoulder" that weight.

Most of us don't realize how hunched over we are from traveling in cars and airplanes and carrying backpacks. People tend to think that this affects only the elderly, but that's not the case. Unless you do something to correct this, I guarantee that you will soon have rotator cuff, back, and neck problems, which will limit your ability to perform.

Our natural instinct is to drop the shoulders forward, especially after long periods of sitting or carrying a backpack. But you ought to do the opposite: Elevate your sternum and let your shoulder blades hang back and down, which will give you proper posture. Imagine yourself feeling tall, as if there's a fishhook inserted under the sternum, pulling you up.

Most athletes have experienced shoulder pain, especially in the front of the shoulder near the groove where the bicep inserts into the shoulder. The problem is an immobile thoracic spine and poor alignment between the rib cage and the pelvis, which causes dysfunctional movement patterns and affects everything connected to that area. Thoracic spine function, therefore, is the foundation to long-term shoulder health.

Many people try to fix the shoulder when they should be addressing a thoracic spine that's out of alignment because of poor posture. This is especially true in younger populations and in tactical athletes from carrying packs and wearing helmets for miles and miles.

The movements in this program will require you to bring your shoulders back and down, but you'll want to make it a daily habit. To make lasting change, you must lengthen your internal rotators (chest and lats) and strengthen the external rotators (the muscles of the upper back, rotator cuff, and the rest of the shoulders).

Summary: Hip, torso (or core), and shoulder stability give us pillar strength, a center axis from which to move. Traditional training programs think of warm-ups in terms of activating the legs or arms. But since movement starts from the pillar, it makes sense instead to first warm up the pillar. That's the role of Pillar Prep, the activation of your shoulders, torso, and hips.

Summary: Pillar Prep is a brief series of movements that activates and strengthens the pillar, giving our body great stability and efficiency prior to doing other movement patterns that rely on the pillar as the foundation. We want to make sure everything is turned on and activated before going through any further movement. By activating the shoulders, torso, and hips, you'll be much better prepared to go through the other units in your training session. Pillar Prep sets the physiological and psychological stage to incorporate pillar strength into every movement of your workout, since every exercise or movement pattern requires it. Pillar Prep allows us to spend a few focused minutes getting our minds and muscles tuned before progressing to other parts of the training program.

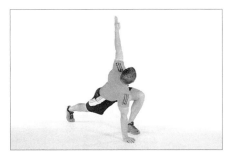

2 | Movement Prep

Movement Preparation has changed the face of sport, decreasing injury while improving the performance of athletes globally.

Movement Prep, which I've used with elite athletes for more than two decades, is an active series of warm-up exercises that efficiently increases the core temperature; activates the nervous system; lengthens, strengthens, stabilizes, and balances muscles; and, as the name suggests, prepares you for the upcoming movements.

The traditional approach to warming up consists of stretch-and-hold static stretching and a general warm-up, such as riding a stationary bike. We want to make this time more efficient by preparing for the movements you're about to undertake. (Static stretching, while not ideal before a workout, is a great option to enhance your flexibility *after* a workout.)

The goal is to improve the long-term mobility and flexibility of your muscles. Rather than have them stretch and revert to where they were—as is the case with stretch-and-hold routines—you want your body to remember these new ranges of motion. This is done through a process of lengthening the muscle (known as active elongation), which is more effective than a traditional stretch. Here's the difference: You don't just passively lengthen your muscles; you actively lengthen and immediately strengthen them by contracting efficiently through this new range of motion. So instead of traditional stretching, you're showing your muscles how to use the motion.

This philosophy is especially important for tactical athletes. If you've spent hours packed in an aircraft or vehicle and suddenly have to jump out and be explosive with both your movement and your decisions, having this foundation of movement quality protects you from risk when operating in this dangerous environment.

Movement Prep is a powerful self-evaluation tool. As you master the movement patterns, pay attention to your posture and pillar strength. Also be aware of any asymmetries between your right and left sides, as well as your front and back. As you get deeper into this program, Movement Prep will be a daily diagnostic of where your body is and will focus you on areas you need to address.

What people fail to realize is that *every* movement, including the time spent warming up, is a self-evaluation that reveals the source of any pain, instability, lack of mobility, and asymmetry in the body. The Movement Prep routine represents the fundamental movement patterns that you must do well as a human and, more important, as a high-performing athlete.

Movement Prep packs a lot of punch into time you previously thought of as just a low-impact warm-up. Movement Prep might look like a combination of active Pilates and yoga blended together in a fluid, integrated way. That's true, but it also will activate all of the small stabilizing muscles in your body that assist with balance. You'll revisit and rekindle all of the proper movement patterns you learned as an infant. That's because Movement Prep is engineered from the software that was ingrained in you when you came out of the womb.

Summary: Movement Prep, which we've used with elite athletes for more than two decades, is an active series of warm-up exercises that efficiently increases the core temperature; activates the nervous system; lengthens, strengthens, stabilizes, and balances muscles; and prepares you for more challenging movements in your training session. Movement Prep will reestablish the mobility, coordination, and joint stability you enjoyed in your younger years and improve your strength, balance, and coordination—in other words, it will heighten your body's ability to process information.

Movement Prep will be a challenge at first. Just remember that the top champions in sports have struggled with it just as much. Like you, they shared the mindset that they soon would master it.

3 | Plyometrics

Plyometrics are movements designed to link strength and speed. These dynamic exercises—up and down, side to side, and twisting back and forth—activate your body's central nervous system, stimulating the fast-twitch muscle fibers so that you can generate force as quickly and efficiently as needed. Movements will include jumps, hops, and bounds in various planes of movement and of various speeds and loads.

Plyos are classified as jumps, bounds, or hops. Jumps are a two-leg takeoff followed by a two-leg landing. Bounds are a one-leg takeoff followed by the opposite one-leg landing. Hops are a one-leg takeoff followed by the same one-leg or two-leg landing.

Plyos are any movement that uses the stretch-shortening cycle (SSC), a rapid muscle lengthening followed immediately by a rapid muscle shortening. Think in terms of placing one hand on the table. Reach over with the other hand, pull a finger back rapidly and let go; you'll hear a powerful snap it as it hits the table. The SSC uses the stretch reflex and stored elastic energy to produce greater power during movement.

Think of the body as a pogo stick, storing and releasing energy powerfully. Plyos improve the ability to coordinate movements, especially changes of direction. By storing and releasing elastic energy, you create far greater speed and power while decreasing the energy expended and improving endurance.

Every movement has some elastic component. Your body, specifically around your fascial and muscular system, has elastic properties. So it's fair to say that you can view your body as a series of rubber bands, strung through your various planes and slings, stretched across the proper joint angles.

To stretch a rubber band, you need to stabilize one end of the band, say, on your thumb, and pull back the other end, as if shooting it across the room. In our program, we focus on the power of stability. The stability is simply the anchor point for your muscles and fascia that allows you to stretch those rubber bands and slings to release a powerful amount of energy.

When the body starts to move, it stretches the opposite/antagonist muscle, storing this potential energy and then ultimately delivering that force in the desired direction. Elasticity does not require large muscular size. It is about the tone or the tension of your muscular and fascial slings as they're pulled from their set point. It stretches them, which allows them to snap back. The speed or the rate of the stretch and the spring of the tension are correlated to how rapidly you will apply force and recover.

The great thing about elasticity is that it doesn't just help you jump higher or run faster. It enables you to move more efficiently. Our goal with this training program is to compress the contractile mechanism of the muscle to allow you to store and release energy in less time, with greater power.

> **Remember:** The more dynamic the exercise, the more elasticity comes into play. The slower the movement, the greater the focus on stability and strength.

Plyos enhance power, but they're also one of the greatest protectors an athlete can have. Elasticity helps you withstand the rapid loads and lengthening of muscle tissue that happens on every stride and play of your sport. If you ever watch athletes go up high for a catch or a dunk and land with their limbs swinging and rolling and wonder how they don't get hurt, thank the elastic system. The body's ability to feel the rate of stretch, store the energy, and return it to the starting point is the saving grace. The next time you see an athlete struck in football or hockey, consider how much outside force is applied to that system and how the body absorbs that force. That's all because of the elastic system. Elasticity gives athletes a set of involuntary brakes and deceleration mechanisms to withstand these high and rapid stretch loads so that the body doesn't disassemble.

Your joints provide the structure of your body, but it's the elastic properties of your muscular fascial system that keep everything connected.

The movements in this unit fall into four categories: rapid, short, long, and very long response.

Rapid-response drills are short, quick movements that improve tissue tolerance. These are low-force, high-speed activities designed to improve your ground reaction forces and quickness.

Short-response drills are high-force, lower frequency movements, such as box blasts, tuck jumps, and hurdle hops. They help you hit the ground and immediately spring back off, improving your body's elasticity. These have the highest rate of force over the shortest range of motion, which is why they're classified as advanced plyometrics.

Long-response drills are moderate-force, longer range of motion movements that focus on stability and power while laying the foundation for more explosive movements. Your feet will stay on the ground longer, but you'll produce higher levels of power with each repetition.

Very long response drills have a longer range of motion and can involve a high degree of force. These can include resisted squat jumps and split jumps with bungee cords or weight vests. We are starting to move into a power training direction here, as this is the start to external loading.

The key with plyometrics is to be fully engaged and apply the maximum amount of force to each rep. As we improve our training, this will become more of a reflex to your body than it will for your brain. It will be all reaction for competition.

Summary: Through plyometrics, you can improve your body's elasticity, its ability to generate and reduce force. By doing so, you'll make it more elastic and springy. Elasticity decreases the potential for injury and allows you to produce more force (or less, if needed) in less time. Plyometrics are the perfect blend of stability, mobility, strength, power, and dynamic balance.

4 | Movement Skills

One of the key philosophies taught at our training centers since our founding in 1999 is the concept of Movement Skills. Yet we've never drilled deep into this concept in our previous books.

Of course, we're all about movement, and the entire program emphasizes creating pillar strength so that we have stability, mobility, and elasticity throughout our bodies to create ideal movement and high performance.

Movement patterns are skills we learned as infants. Remember the child we talked about earlier, learning to move with a forearm commando crawl and progressing to crawling on the hands and finally to pulling himself upright? Those are skills. Every sport or tactical athlete has a specific set of movement skills that must be mastered in order for that athlete to move as efficiently as possible with the least amount of energy wasted.

In this part of the program, we focus on two areas of movement: linear and multidirectional.

Linear movement skill training refers to developing the technique and power required to project the body in one direction. Linear movement can be broken into start, acceleration, transition, and absolute speed mechanics. Acceleration refers to building velocity from a stationary position and changing power or direction—think zero to 15 yards. Absolute speed refers to the mechanics required to maintain velocity over distance. This involves top-end speed. Think about making efficient gear changes in a race car. You know you will kill the engine or jerk down the road if you try moving straight from first to fifth gear. The body reacts the same way if you put yourself in an inefficient position to generate speed and ultimately exhaust your mechanics. These movement skills specific to your sport are what you're trying to improve for speed, power, and endurance.

Movement Skills represent your ability to apply the highest speed at the right time with the right angle of force into the ground or something else. Some might consider Movement Skills speed training, and indeed that's part of it. But we don't call this process "Movement Skills" just to give it a catchy name; we do it to drive awareness that there is skill required to be fast and efficient so you can express speed and power whenever it's needed.

With Movement Skills, we'll focus on the various angles that help you generate power between your foot and shin, between shin and thigh, between thigh and pillar, and all of this in relationship to the ground. You're going to accelerate, decelerate, store energy, and reaccelerate. What you'll notice within the drills in this unit is they bring together and improve all your mobility, stability, speed, and power to take your movement skills to the next level. This program will make you faster and more powerful—for a longer period of time.

Most athletes who arrive at our facilities think their movement skills are quite good. Some believe that by improving stability and flexibility, they'll get faster. Do more strength training, take the right supplements, and do high-speed interval workouts, and you'll get faster.

There's some truth to that, of course, and all of those elements are part of this system. But unless you first focus on movement skills, you're going to have a difficult time maximizing the results from your efforts in those other areas.

Let's take absolute speed. That's a movement skill, not just natural ability or genetics. We pride ourselves on making athletes faster, regardless of size or age. When you train to strike the ground properly with the foot to propel the hips forward from a tall, upright position, your absolute speed will improve. We do this by actual movement drills that break down sprinting into its various components.

Movement Skills produce aha moments with athletes when they realize how the movements directly correlate to their sport. It's like in the movie *The Karate Kid* when Daniel realized that all those hours spent painting Mr. Miyagi's fences and waxing his cars actually were helping him perfect the movements necessary to thrive in karate. Unfortunately, our athletes aren't sprucing up our facilities with this training, but they sure make it look great when they execute the movements learned within our walls.

This is what puts everything together for our athletes. Terms such as *stability*, *mobility*, *elasticity*, *relative power*, and *endurance* will resonate in your competitive field, whether it's in sport or the tactical space. This is why you do what you do.

Our Movement Skills universe is vast and exceeds the constraints of this book, though we encourage you to dig deeper at www.coreperformance.com. Our goal here is to give you high-impact movement skills that can be done in the smallest of spaces and directly correlate to your on-field performance.

Whatever kind of athlete you are, you will benefit from learning how to better apply force and cut with greater speed and agility to separate from the defender or to close on the elusive opponent. The same holds true in the tactical environment, where we break down all movement patterns to, say, cross streets at maximum speed in hostile environments while the shoulders are turned downrange, firing accurately.

Movement skills are much like the blocks in a masonry wall. Consider the 40-yard dash, made famous by the NFL Combine. We've trained hundreds of NFL hopefuls to link their stance, start, acceleration, and transition to improve the key movement skill of absolute speed. How efficiently we link these skills together and transition from one to the next determines success.

We take these movement skills and bring them together for very sport-specific tasks. Think about a wide receiver running a route. There's the movement skill of a two-point stance, the start, acceleration, deceleration, cut, reacceleration, catch, and deceleration before the sideline. That's a specific football movement—a 15-yard out pattern—but the movement skills apply to whatever athletic endeavor you choose.

The key to movement skills is being able to deliver them when called upon. Practicing these skills will provide only a modest return if we haven't first mastered the underlying movement patterns. For example, if an athlete has chronic ankle issues and does not have proper ankle mobility to glide the shin and knee over the foot, he will not be able to execute the movement properly. If the ankle is locked at a 90-degree angle, then we will never get the body in the right position, let alone stretch those muscles.

With the ankle locked, the athlete cannot cut or accelerate. Other areas will compensate, which will place undue stress on those muscles and joints. It's a vicious cycle, but one we can nip in the bud. By mastering Pillar Prep and Movement Prep, we'll create the foundation that allows us to execute Movement Skills.

Putting Your Best Feet Forward

Minimalist athletic footwear is one of the more popular footwear trends of recent years. It can be a valuable strategy to boost your performance so long as it's applied properly.

The greatest percentage of sensory input receptors can be found in the foot. Of the body's 206 bones, 25 percent are in the feet. The human foot has 28 bones, 33 joints, 107 ligaments, and 19 tendons. This means there's tremendous value to training with your feet as close to the ground as possible. It improves tissue quality and leg strength while helping you recover from wearing other footwear.

Step down gradually. Go from a traditional stability shoe to a performance trainer to "barefoot" shoes. Give yourself at least several weeks to let your movement patterns adapt.

Start with a morning routine of rolling your feet one at a time for thirty seconds on a baseball, tennis ball, or golf ball. Balancing on one foot turns on the hip stabilizers, while rolling the ball in your arch releases the fascia and activates the various trigger points in the foot. It also reinforces the importance of the big toe.

This gets you out of your shoes and rolling over that big toe, which most people aren't accustomed to. The big toe is the trigger to the whole kinetic chain. That's why if people are walking, we want them walking with their feet straight ahead, rolling over the big toe.

Many newcomers to toe shoes complain that it's difficult to spread their toes apart sufficiently to slip into the shoes quickly. That's the fault of the user, not the shoe. You should be able to extend the toes and slide them right in. How quickly you can put on these shoes demonstrates the level of dexterity and motor control you have.

Think of this as phalangeal fitness. We should be able to separate our toes as easily as we do our fingers. But years of wearing shoes condition our feet otherwise. The solution? Take off your shoes and socks regularly and work on moving your toes apart from one another.

With minimalist shoes, the feet should contact the ground underneath the hips, producing a more efficient transfer of energy through the body. Stride length becomes shorter and more compact. The feet respond by naturally increasing the arch strength of the foot.

Think of that arch like a spring. If you have a nice arch, when your foot hits the ground, the arch expands like a spring and snaps back. That's the goal of the arch—to store and release energy. It lengthens and snaps back. In normal shoes, we lose a lot of these dynamics.

It's normal to have some soreness when transitioning to minimalist footwear, but stop if you're having any pain. Do arch rolls on a tennis ball, baseball, or golf ball before and after training with minimalist footwear and use a soft tissue massage stick on your calves. Foot hygiene is always important, but especially when shifting to minimalist footwear. Look for cuts or breaks in the skin, calluses, and blisters. Keep toenails trimmed and neat. Wearing minimalist footwear makes you more prone to ingrown toenails, which can be as debilitating as turf toe or an ankle injury.

People don't take care of their feet, especially guys. Taking care of your feet is important if you're going to experience the benefits of training with a minimalist shoe.

Incorporating minimalist footwear can provide numerous benefits. Start with wearing them for Pillar Prep, Movement Prep, and Recovery workouts and you should see immediate results.

LINEAR MOVEMENT

Linear movement is the ability to transfer force at a high rate of speed. It is broken into four components: the start, acceleration, the transition, and absolute speed.

At the start, establish a balanced position where your center of gravity is as high as possible and in front of the base of support. Picture top sprinters. They're not hunched over; they're standing tall, but leaning slightly forward. This enables them to maximize force into the ground from head to heel in a controlled manner with the greatest possible velocity.

At the start, the lower body should be in the triple flexion position. The feet are hip-width apart in a staggered position. The ankle should be dorsiflexed (toes up) as much as possible, producing an angle of about 45 degrees to the shin. You

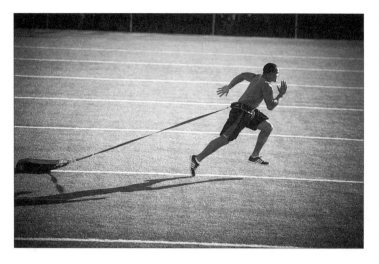

should be looking 10 yards ahead. The elbows should be flexed at 90 degrees, working in a motion from hand to hip, and from hand to head.

Acceleration has to do with your start, whether that's a fixed-position track start, a two-point stance, or accelerating from a position common to your sport. Acceleration lasts from zero to 15 yards. After that, we transition into absolute speed, which is where your body is much more upright and your leg action is more cyclical. Between your arm and leg action, you're feeling like you're running from the center of your body in a fluid motion. This allows you to hit your peak or top-end speed and sustain this rate. This can last from yard 15 to 20 through the rest of your race, whether that's a 50-yard sprint or hundreds of yards.

The benefit of acceleration is that as you're forced into longer distances, the same mechanics make your running more efficient, boosting speed while decreasing the effort needed.

As you accelerate, push off both feet and get full extension through your hips, knees, and ankles. This maximizes the force into the ground, transfers force throughout the body, and brings as much power as possible to the acceleration. When accelerating, lean forward about 45 degrees, maintaining a straight line from your ankle through the hips, torso, and neck. Think in terms of feeling tall through your pillar.

The legs should drive ahead in a pistonlike motion, as if they're attacking the ground with each step. You should be flexing one hip while keeping the other fully extended. (By mastering Pillar Prep and Movement Prep, you will make this possible.)

As the foot leaves the ground, the leg enters into the swing phase, where you have triple flexion of the hip (90 degrees), knee (less than 90), and ankle (fully dorsiflexed). The key to staying in this position is keeping the toe up (or dorsiflexed), which is one of the most important elements of running mechanics.

Upper-body mechanics also play a key role in acceleration, as you want to transfer energy from the upper body to the lower body through your powerful pillar. Maintain a stiff pillar position, but use your arms. When you don't use your arms, you don't fully engage the power of your pillar. Your torso and legs alone can't fully use this efficient storing and releasing of elastic energy critical to taking your performance to the next level.

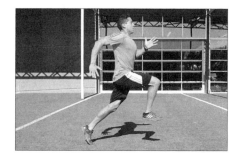

ABSOLUTE SPEED AND RUNNING ECONOMY

By using your arms and shoulders effectively, you actually create and "recycle" more energy. You do this by relaxing the shoulders and keeping your arms bent at roughly 90 degrees, as if your hands were constantly going from your back pockets to your nose. With your elbows driving back and forth along your torso, your chest and the front of your shoulders and torso can stretch. Your elbows naturally will snap back to the front of your body, creating an efficient pendulumlike motion.

What does this have to do with acceleration? In a word: everything. Human movement is integrated; you'll find that your arm action dictates your leg action.

In order to have great linear movement and acceleration, you must have the full range of motion. After relative power (more on that shortly), mobility is the key to acceleration and linking the upper and lower body. If you have restrictions in your shoulders, for instance, it will affect your ability to maintain a strong pillar while generating force with the arms. If you're lacking in hip and knee mobility, it will affect your ability to extend fully. A lack of ankle mobility will make it difficult to create the dorsiflexion that's crucial to efficient running mechanics.

MULTIDIRECTIONAL SPEED

Multidirectional speed is the key to most sports, as well as thriving in a battle environment. To improve your multidirectional speed, it's necessary to approach it like any complex skill by breaking it down into individual components.

We start the teaching progressions in a basic stance, which is what basketball

The Power of Dorsiflexion

Grab a partner and take this simple test to see how well you dorsiflex. Lie facedown on the ground and pull one leg up, as if performing a leg curl. Try to hold your leg at a 90-degree angle to the floor, as if in the middle of a leg curl, and have your partner try to pull your foot back toward the ground. Don't let your partner move it. You'll notice that your hamstring will fire, and for most people, the toe will pull up toward the shin and two big muscles will pop from the back of your calf.

Now assume the same position, your leg again at a 90-degree angle to the floor. Point your toe up toward the ceiling and have your partner hold it there. Then have your partner try to pull down on the heel. You'll be surprised to find that the tension on the hamstring is twice as much and that the calf muscle is shut off and mushy.

Why does this matter? Because your leg goes through this action with every stride you take. If your toe is down, your calf is shut off, and your hamstring will have to do twice the work than if your calf was turned on or activated, as it is when your toe is up. With your toe down, you'll experience greater hamstring fatigue, which places an increased load on the tissues and causes slower and lower performance. You'll also be exposed to chronic hamstring tightness, which will lead to hamstring injuries.

How the foot strikes the ground often confuses runners. Some try to strike with the heel. Others try to run on the toes. Neither is correct. With proper dorsiflexion, your stride's strike zone is beneath your hip, not out in front of your body. This way, you create a straight line from ear to ankle.

players know as the triple-threat position: feet just wider than shoulder-width apart, knees bent at 90 degrees for a strong base of support.

If you have a partner, have him or her try to push you over sideways at the hips, then move up to your ribs, then push hard on your shoulders. You'll immediately feel the right posture and "angles" you need to have. You might also experience one of those aha, *Karate Kid*–type moments where you realize how valuable all that work was to build pillar strength.

From this balanced, triple-threat position, you can step laterally, slide, go into a crossover move or a drop step, jump, accelerate, or transition between any of them. You'll master each one of these units and link them together through

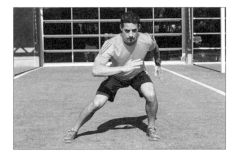

drills, discovering improved coordination, speed, and power while moving more efficiently.

Next we'll introduce random agility, the ability to react and move when faced with an outside stimulus. Random agility usually is tested in the field of sport or battle. We will give you some concepts that make up the majority of multidirectional movement. If you can master lateral and base cutting, as well as a powerful crossover step, you will have a strong multidirectional foundation. This, combined with acceleration, gives you the ability to have great multidirectional speed.

Lateral and base position is the foundation to most athletic movement. Think about when you learned how to throw a ball or fire a gun. You began with great pillar strength, with your feet outside the hips, bending at the ankle and knee. You leaned slightly forward at the hips, placing yourself in a balanced and powerful position.

When you're in this position, your weight should feel like it's on your midfoot to the ball of your foot, slightly shifted forward. From the side view we should be able to see angles between the foot and shin, the shin and thigh, and the thigh and pillar. In this position, you should feel balanced to move forward or laterally, drop step, or jump. You should be ready for anything that your opponent can throw at you.

This is the lateral and base position. This is the position you will start from or transition into before you move right or left or have to return backward. Almost everyone starts and finishes with this lateral and base in most athletic activities. This position allows your body to have great dynamic balance—as defined by keeping your pillar inside your base of support.

The reason we're so adamant about establishing pillar strength is that it leads into using lateral and base actively, which is known as cutting. Cutting is rapidly decelerating the body by planting the foot, keeping the body inside the base of support, and then moving in a different direction. Imagine yourself moving toward the right, planting your right foot, and cutting back toward your left while avoiding an opponent or an object. That might sound simple; perhaps it's something you've done many times. But it's rarely done correctly. That's because most athletes we see lack ankle and/or hip mobility on one side or the other. So it's physically impossible for them to create the proper angles and stretch the right muscles to cut properly. Plus, most athletes don't have enough pillar strength. When they place one foot on the ground, the shoulders and pillar continue to move toward that outside cut, moving the chest and shoulder over the foot. They don't have enough pillar strength to decelerate their pillar and keep it inside the base of support. Not only does this lead to poor performance, it puts you at major risk for injuries of the ankles, hips, and especially the knees. Now let's compound this by adding an opponent who is pushing you, adding significantly more force to your body.

Once you've mastered these movement patterns, you will be an efficient, elastic athlete who can store these rapid-force loads and release that energy in the opposite direction with greater speed and power, which actually requires less effort.

When we cut, we can't forget the inside leg, which plays a significant role in deceleration. This inside leg should remain outside your base of support to help slow you down and be there as a backup in case your outside cutting foot were to give way. The inside leg would catch your weight and allow you to move back in the other direction.

Most people have poor lateral movement patterns that cause them to be slow and more prone to tightness and injury, especially in the groin area. Many sports coaches have taught players to slide laterally by, say, reaching out with the left or lead leg and foot, pointing toward the left. That's a dangerous move, because when the leg is externally rotated and pointed away, you have no ability to cut and plant in the opposite direction from that foot.

Remember: The lateral and base position has both feet straight ahead perpendicular to the hips, which allows you to push and cut from the inside of the foot. When you rotate the foot out, you lose this ability. When you try to stop, your foot moves forward toward the front of your shoe. Your knee slides forward over the shin to try to go over the shoe, causing sheer forces on your knee, leading to greater potential for injury.

Make sure that both toes point straight ahead. Push off the back leg and be sure to keep your feet apart in that lateral base so that your torso and pillar stay within that base of support, allowing you to move in any direction that the situation requires: forward, drop step back, back the opposite direction, or planting and going vertical.

In order to improve these multidirectional skills, knowing that many athletes are confined to inside spaces during winter months or at home, we've picked a few drills that don't take a lot of space. We will place these in your movement work-outs. We'll also be using shuttle runs, since they force you to improve these move-ment patterns while using more energy. This is what makes most court and team sport athletes fatigued more so than just their cardiovascular capacity.

For one movement, we'll place an agility belt around your waist. If you're not in the proper lateral and base position, you might get pulled over. After doing that once, you'll automatically assume the proper position, much like you felt when your partner was pushing on you. As you work with the resistance returning you back from where you came, you'll be pulled at a greater rate of speed, increasing the forces as you decelerate, which will improve your overall elasticity, power, and body position.

We'll also do a lateral bound with a miniband that will show you how to gener-ate power pushing laterally, but also how to stabilize on an outside leg, absorbing with your hips, knees, and ankle with great stability while keeping the opposite leg away, maintaining your base as you will when you cut.

The other key movement pattern in multidirectional speed is the crossover. The easiest way to envision this is to think about the Heisman Trophy. If you're moving laterally to your left and you want to sprint to your left, you need to turn your shoulders and hips in the direction you want to go and rapidly get into an ac-celeration pattern. The crossover allows you to cover a great distance in a power-ful stride.

The key to a great crossover step is to imagine yourself cutting from the right leg within your base of support. As you press off the outside leg, the inside leg pulls the hips in the direction you'd like to go (internal hip rotation). As you push off the outside leg, you should have the same types of mechanics as in acceleration: knees, heels, and toes driving in the direction you want to go, and ready to power-fully attack the ground from effective angles.

Multidirectional speed is hard work, which is why coaches call it hustle. You need relative power, efficiency, endurance, and work ethic to become effective at it. Multidirectional speed requires all these motor abilities working together, including the most important one, which is your relentless drive to be quick and powerful from the start all the way to the finish.

SUMMARY: Through Movement Skills training, we're going to reestablish and perfect the fundamental movements that we learned as infants, then practice specific athletic skills through focusing on linear and multidirectional speed. By breaking down our movements into learnable segments, we'll become faster while moving with greater efficiency and with reduced potential for injury.

5 | Medicine Ball

The medicine ball has thousands of years of credibility as a tool to develop mobility, stability, and especially power.

But the medicine ball is more than just a powerful tool in an athlete's arsenal; it's an entire unit of this program. We're going to use med balls to improve our relative power and elasticity, bridging the gap between strength and speed by using them in various explosive forms.

Your job is to wear out the med ball, trying to break it open. Some of the drills

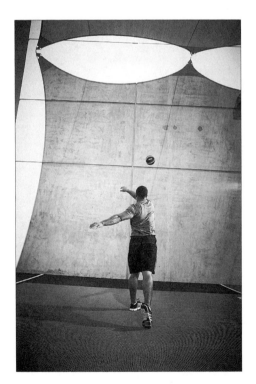

will be familiar movements from the weight room, but the great thing about the balls is that we can use them in a rapid dynamic or ballistic fashion. When we perform, say, a squat press to throw, we're getting the added benefit of being able to release the weighted object. Not only that, but med ball drills are an effective, fun routine. With just a ball and a wall, you can let out all of your frustrations with great elasticity, power, and endurance across all movement patterns.

We're going to take that ball and do rapid chest presses, along with overhead and rotational movements. You'll develop the power to throw, swing, or strike with tremendous force. We'll also take the ball and unleash our power with various types of slams into the wall or into the ground.

All of this will improve your kinetic linking. This is a fancy term for the body's ability to transfer energy from one segment to another. Think of how golfers generate power from their feet, through the hips, shoulders, arms, and hands, ultimately to the club.

This type of powerful transfer of energy can also be

seen in martial arts. As with golf, it has nothing to do with the size of the athlete. Think of Bruce Lee, small in size but massive when it came to producing massive power through efficient movement. From a balanced stance, he could slightly coil, harnessing amazing energy that he redirected toward his target. This is a perfect example of what we want to do with almost every competitive movement.

With med balls, as with any equipment, picking the right ball is important. We want a rubber ball weighing between 6 and 12 pounds. There are heavier balls, but let's start with this size. As you throw the ball against the wall, you'll deal with both the weight and the speed with which it returns from the wall. The more air pressure, the more rapidly it will return off the wall. That creates greater forces for you to decelerate and reaccelerate into the wall, increasing the intensity of the movement. So not only will we progress the number of sets and reps, we'll add to the intensity with increased air pressure.

Early in your med ball training, you'll want to lessen the air pressure so the ball does not rebound as rapidly. This will allow you to master the timing and coordination of the movement. As you get more adept at throwing and catching the ball, increase the air pressure gradually.

There are infinite ways to use the med ball, and we're going to start with movements calling on you to hold the ball as you go through specific movement patterns, accelerating and decelerating the ball as you go. This will help you acquire the ability to store and release elastic energy using your tuned kinetic linking.

Elasticity translates into power and is not a function of muscle size. Elasticity is a function of your ability to store and release energy in a highly coordinated effort within your muscles individually and between them collectively to produce efficient movement. Our goal is to build your body to produce elastic power more efficiently, while protecting it from short-term pain and long-term ailments.

The medicine ball reinforces your strong pillar position because the ball weighs just enough that if you're slightly out of balance, unstable, or in poor alignment, you'll feel awkward and not very powerful. That's a direct biofeedback mechanism that will prompt you to get back in the proper position.

As you progress, you'll be ready to generate greater power by doing more ballistic and dynamic throws. To perform these movements, find a solid, flat surface, preferably a concrete or block wall—any place where you can throw and catch a medicine ball. At EXOS, we've become connoisseurs of med balls, and we feature a number of different balls that are more or less likely to bounce.

When performing these movements, pay close attention to the position of your hands. Your lead hand—the one closest to the wall—should stay under the ball. Your back hand is perpendicular to the lead hand and touches it, pinkie to pinkie. That creates a cup for the ball to sit in and allows you to guide it through the range of motion. Initiate the movement from your feet and transfer force through your hips, torso, and shoulders into your hands. This will improve kinetic efficiency and develop more power than just throwing the ball with your arms alone.

You'll likely find, as many of our athletes do, that the Medicine Ball unit becomes one of your favorites.

SUMMARY: The medicine ball is much more than a piece of training equipment that has stood the test of time. It's a key unit of the Athletes' Performance Training System that will help you master fundamental movement patterns while generating power across all three planes of motion.

6 | Relative Power

Power = Strength/Time

Power is strength divided by time. Relative power reflects your power-to-weight ratio. If a 175-pound athlete drops to 160 pounds but maintains the same power and strength, his relative power has gone through the roof.

Relative power makes the most efficient athlete. The term *relative* means "per pound," so we want to create the most efficient athlete per pound. In other industries this is called the power-to-weight ratio. Most of the fun things in life—cars, planes, motorcycles, etc.—have special power-to-weight ratios.

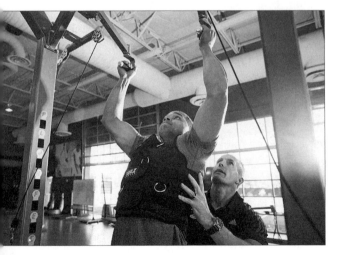

Relative power makes things easier for the athlete. He's better able to control that body weight and also to efficiently decelerate it and reaccelerate it into the ground or someone else. Power is strength on demand, getting you what you want faster and easier.

By using the word *power*, we are factoring in the concept of per unit time. When we start talking about athletes in sport and their ability to execute, everything is in per unit time. That's what wins races. That's the difference in one wide receiver stopping on a dime and quickly cutting the other way versus another player with lesser power making a long, laborious cut. One gets away from his defender and makes the catch while the other remains covered.

There is a misconception that in order to become powerful you need larger muscles or more weight. If we have an athlete weighing 200 pounds with 10 percent body fat, he has roughly 180 pounds of lean mass and 20 pounds of body fat. Let's say we keep him at 10 percent body fat but we add 10 pounds of lean body mass. Now let's measure his before and after performance in the vertical jump, which along with the broad jump is one of the two main tests of relative power. If his performance remained the same, most coaches and scientists would see that as a huge positive. After all, he was able to gain 10 pounds and still jump as high. His average and peak power output, according to that mindset, has significantly improved.

At EXOS, I would say we failed. Our expectation with the way that we train for power is that if we add 10 pounds of lean body mass, we expect his vertical jump to improve and for him to become faster. We didn't just add lean body mass with the same power profile. Instead, we created greater relative power within his existing mass.

That's our goal when we talk about relative power.

People often assume that more lean body mass is better. That's not so for the majority of sports that are not combative or position-dominant games. With most sports, adding lean body mass just for the sake of adding lean body mass probably will make the body *less* efficient. You've added more overall mass to carry, and depending on where that mass is distributed, it could force you to work that much harder to accelerate and decelerate with every stride you take.

We want to decrease your body fat while maintaining and improving the efficiency of your lean body mass. "Intelligent" lean mass is more valuable than massive bodybuilder muscle because it possesses greater mobility, stability, movement patterns, power, strength, and endurance. Bodybuilder muscle is all for show. Intelligent lean mass is for go.

In the Relative Power unit, we'll alternate between pushing movements (upper and lower body), pulling movements (upper and lower body), and rotational movements.

As with everything in this program, this accomplishes more in the least amount of time. If we do an upper-body press exercise, the muscles become fatigued. That's a good thing, of course. Now if we follow that up immediately with an upper-body or lower-body pull exercise, we're allowing those muscles that performed the upper-body press to rest briefly.

If we go right into an opposing exercise, like the upper push to upper pull above, these opposite or antagonistic movements will cause the muscle groups to experience reciprocal inhibition, which promotes the muscle's recovery. So we've improved the quality and efficiency of the program and will get results faster.

Not only that, but we're increasing our workout density, the amount of work per unit time. We're not resting, just alternating movements to make the most of our time and stimulating positive hormone-releasing activities. If you've spent time in a gym, you've probably noticed people who do one set of an exercise, then wait between one to five minutes before attempting another set of the same movement. By training more efficiently, we're working in the cardiovascular system as well as the muscular system. Much like interval training, this will stress the body and stimulate its adaptation to stress while decreasing body fat, increasing caloric expenditure, and improving overall performance levels for hours and days after the workout.

You'll gain power and strength as we continually challenge you by increasing the number of sets and/or repetitions, by increasing the resistance, and also by adjusting the tempo in which you perform each rep.

Tempo simply refers to the cadence in which you go through each movement pattern. An example of this would be if I give you a cadence of 3-2-1, you will lower the weight in three seconds, pause at the isometric position for two seconds, and then press the weight up in one second, hence a 3-2-1 tempo for eccentric (lowering), isometric (bottom), and concentric (raising) contractions.

It's important to remember that injuries often occur when we are tired, whether in sports or daily life. Conditioning is not just a function of your lungs, but possessing efficient movement patterns, greater relative power, strength (pound for pound), and elasticity allows the body to bounce back from fatigue faster.

SUMMARY: Power is strength divided by time. Relative power reflects your power-to-weight ratio. The athlete who can produce the greatest power per pound of body weight has the best relative power.

7 | Energy Systems Development (ESD)

There's nothing wrong with the terms *cardio* or *cardiovascular*, which mean "of, relating to, or involving the heart and the blood vessels." Unfortunately, it's come to be associated with long, slow, inefficient training. The idea of slow, steady-state training for the purposes of losing weight by burning more calories in your "fat-burning zone" is not only a waste of time, but a losing battle if there ever was one.

Cardio exercise traditionally has been considered a means to an end, typically weight loss or fat burning. We need to view it as the means to creating more power. Power is the rate at which you perform work and your ability to maintain high intensities of effort for longer periods of time. This process of creating more power is what we call Energy Systems Development, or ESD.

ESD develops endurance, which allows us to make efficient, high-speed movements for short bursts of time followed by active recovery, followed by additional bursts of movement. You're able to perform at higher intensities repeatedly without becoming fatigued. When everyone on the field is exhausted at the end of a game, you'll be as fresh and as fast as you were at the beginning, giving you a competitive advantage.

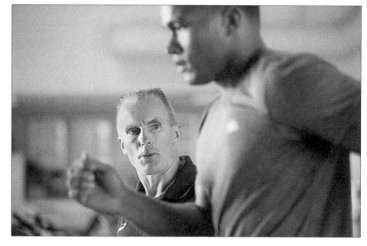

Our goal here is not to lose weight or burn fat, which might occur to some degree, but rather to improve the body's ability to generate and use energy. This won't happen via one long, slow workout that numbs your body and mind and creates repetitive trauma. ESD will require more energy and focus, but less time.

If you are an endurance enthusiast, you might expect to dive into seven different training zones. We will not be doing that in this book. We will use ESD to complement the other work you are doing, and you'll see the synergy of your efforts. Developing your work capacity is a cumulative effect from everything in the Athletes' Performance Training System—from Pillar Prep and Movement Skills to ESD and Regeneration.

We *do* believe in the power of intervals, alternating between periods of work and rest, to develop this endurance. Another benefit of interval training is you'll burn more calories during the session and will continue burning them long after you're done. Instead of doing thirty to sixty minutes of cardio without feeling much impact, now you likely will feel exhausted after fifteen to twenty-five minutes of ESD training. You'll get twice the benefit in half the time.

For your ESD we are going to vary the intensity between sprint, hard, moderate, and easy efforts. This might seem simple, but it is highly effective, and you won't find anything easy about this approach. Feel free to wear a heart rate monitor, watching your response within the rep, during rest intervals, and when repeating (and outperforming) past sessions.

Many training programs use heart rate zones to prescribe the efforts. We will not be using heart rate zones, which are often based off a percentage of your maximal heart rate as calculated with "220 minus your age." This is accurate only 50 percent of the time at best. Instead, we want you focused on the work and effort to achieve faster times or longer distance in the amount of time given, depending on the session.

As your fitness improves, you'll see you are running faster at the same heart rates, showing higher power outputs per heartbeat. This is a powerful concept we call pulse power, which is the embodiment of your overall human system across efficient movement patterns, relative power, and endurance.

In this unit we're going to develop your three energy systems: alactate, lactate, and aerobic. The alactate system boosts your energy from nothing to something for upward of the first twenty seconds, like the first gear in your car, relying on the body's stored energy, not oxygen. Because it doesn't last long, your body needs to shift to the middle gear quickly.

Your body's lactate system refers to its capacity to do high-intensity work and can last up to an hour in very elite athletes. The downside of the lactate system is that your body kicks off lots of waste products faster than it can clear them, which increases your blood pH balance. This is what makes your muscles burn.

For recovery between hard efforts or long-duration, low-intensity efforts, your body is engineered with the efficient aerobic system. The aerobic system runs on stored long-term energy and oxygen to allow us to recover from high-performance work.

Our ESD approach of using intervals of work and recovery is why the more sprints or intervals you do, the more your aerobic system is working. This is why high-intensity training improves both thresholds and VO_2 max, your maximal cardiac output.

Each ESD workout starts with a warm-up period. Then you'll alternate intervals of work with intervals of recovery. You'll do between one and twelve repetitions of this interval, depending on the stage of the program, followed by a cool-down period.

The relationship between the intervals of work and recovery is what we call the work-to-rest ratio. The greater the rest, the higher quality the work should be. The lower the ratio—for instance, one second of work per one second of rest (one to one)—the bigger the challenge, since the body has less time to recover.

You will do the conditioning at the end of several sessions. There is a reason for this, as all of our workouts start with the greatest quality work where the mind and body need to be fresh and focused, and then we work toward more quality endurance, or quantity. This concept can be visualized much like a pyramid, with maximal power at the top and ESD at the bottom. You'll see in the following template explanation that there will be an ESD block at the end of each session. Here is a quick overview of the program, which is integrated into your training templates.

Strength Day ESD			
	Day A	Day B	Day C
Foundational	Lactate Capacity 0:30 Hard/4:30 Moderate	Lactate Power (Long) 1:00 Hard/1:00 Easy	
Power Phases 1 & 3	Lactate Power (Long) 300 Yard Shuffle (≈1:00)	Lactate Power (Short) 150 Yard Ladder Shuttle (≈0:30)	Alactate Power (Long) 100 Yard Sprint (≈0:15)
Power Phases 2 & 4	Lactate Power (Short) 150 Yard Shuttle (≈0:30)	Alactate Power (Long) 60 Yard Ladder Shuttle (≈0:15)	Alactate Power (Short) 50 Yard Sprint (≈0:07)

Movement and Regeneration ESD		
Movement Session Linear/Combo	Movement Session Multidirectional	Regeneration
Lactate Capacity 5:00 Hard/1:00 Easy	Lactate Capacity 0:30 Sprint/4:30 Hard (Track Distance)	Aerobic 20:00 + Easy

In order to get in the greatest shape of your life using the ESD sessions in the program, you need to understand the definitions of how you are asked to execute the training session. We've kept it simple so you can execute this even while fatigued.

Sprint = 90+ percent, as fast as you can go (rate of perceived exertion is a 10/10)
Hard = Very difficult effort, breathing very heavily, cannot speak (nor want to) (RPE 8–9/10)

Moderate = Difficult, breathing heavily, can speak with difficulty (RPE 7–8/10)

Easy = Hard enough to break a sweat, but still able to carry on a conversation (RPE 4–5/10)

In addition to adapting your efforts to the prescribed intensities, you'll need to do some additional work by tracking your results. There are sessions where we prescribe intervals based on distance. When that's the case, keep track of how much time it takes you to complete your reps. As your fitness improves, your times for a given distance should go down. If we give you an interval based on time, track how much distance you are able to cover.

The goal is to have both movement pattern efficiency and maximal power, normally measured by wattage or speed, and to hold this quality over time, or quality endurance. This is not where you check out mentally and physically to achieve a tough goal. Your movement should never look sloppy, even when you are most fatigued. No, this is where elite athletes shine and where novices learn to embrace the moment and make the most out of this performance.

SUMMARY: Unlike traditional cardio work, Energy Systems Development focuses on developing quality-to-quality endurance. You'll develop speed and power, then speed and power endurance, resulting in pulse power. This will require your integrated energy systems (alactate, lactate, and aerobic) to feed the demands you must endure to play at the top of your game, from the first snap or engagement through the last, at the highest quality physically and mentally.

THE ATHLETES' PERFORMANCE WORKOUT: AN INTRODUCTION

We've given you a lot of information thus far and have no doubt you can handle it. Our goal is to provide you with simple solutions that will maximize your return on investment and minimize risk of injury.

How do we do that?

We're going to organize this entire system into three session types: Movement Skills, Power, and Regeneration. There are three Movement Skills sessions. The first is Linear Speed, which enhances acceleration and absolute speed. There's a Multidirectional Speed session focused on cutting, shuffling, and crossover movements. The last one is a Combination workout, which include all aspects of speed. We'll come back to these in a moment.

The Power sessions are organized into five phases, each with a different emphasis. The first time you go through this program you'll progress through the phases linearly, lasting fifteen weeks. Once you have made it through, you will be empowered to use this modular system to customize this to your competition or deployment schedule, which is detailed later.

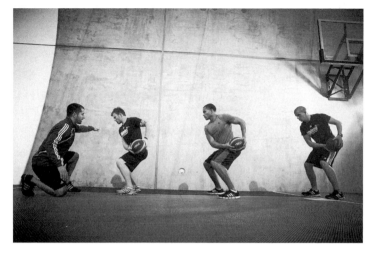

You know Work + Rest = Success, and we've created nine different Regeneration sessions for you to pick from based upon what you may feel you need for that day. You might also incorporate chunks of this daily, first thing in the morning, before or after your training sessions, or in the evening as you decompress.

To effectively move through the book's workout, we're going to first need to understand how to move from phase to phase. After creating this macro view of your plan, or what you are doing from week to week, we'll dial in and create a weekly view of what you will be doing. Once the weekly plan is established, then we'll dive into specifically what you are doing each day.

There are five Power phases to the program: Foundational, and Power 1–4. Each of the five Power phases has specific goals.

The Foundational phase is designed to create a strong foundation for future power development by "cleaning" your movement patterns, removing any asymmetries, and improving mobility and stability. Challenge yourself during this phase and you'll find new levels of strength to build on as a result of these upgrades. This happens for nearly every elite performer we have trained. Go in with a mindset of setting a proper foundation from which to move forward.

The other four phases are labeled Power 1–4. In Power 1, we're going to use isolateral (one limb at a time) and bilateral (two limbs at a time) movements. This will allow us to build your ability to produce force and lay the foundation for greater power later. We'll do this via descending sets, where the reps will decrease week to week. You will increase resistance while attempting to move the weight quickly. So that's fewer reps with increased resistance and intensity.

In Power 1, we'll follow a tempo of 3-0-X. That means we'll take three seconds during the eccentric (lowering) part of the lift. There's no pause before explosively lifting. This maximizes your force development by stimulating intramuscular coordination. If you think explosively, you'll be explosive. In 3-0-X, 3 = 3 seconds down, 0 = no pause in the middle, and X = explosive

The ESD (Energy Systems Development) work in Power 1 will consist of ESD on both the Power days as well as the Movement Skills and Regeneration days. On the first day, you'll do 300-yard shuttles, which will take you around sixty seconds. Track your time for each rep, and if you have a heart rate monitor, you can track how quickly you recover between shuttles. You'll need to compare this against the Power 3 phase.

On the second day, you'll do 150-yard ladder shuttles. A ladder consists of running 5 yards out and back and repeating at distances of 10, 15, 20, and 25 yards, for a total of 150 yards. On the third day, we'll do 100-yard sprints, where we focus on the movement patterns we've refined in this program. On Regeneration days, we do twenty minutes of nonimpact work on a treadmill, stationary bike, swimming, etc.

In Power 2, we'll again do a mix of isolateral and bilateral work. The volume of work will be less, but the intensity greater. We'll do this again by descending sets, further increasing the resistance and the pace. This is the time to challenge yourself both with the amount of resistance and how rapidly you can move the weight. In Power 2, we'll introduce contrasting, a combination of strength and plyos to increase the rate of force development and elasticity.

You will do a strength exercise to get the maximal recruitment from your muscles immediately followed by a similar movement in a plyometric or elastic fashion so that we can move with greater speed and elasticity. This links speed and strength, creating power.

In Power 2, we'll speed up the tempo to 1-0-X. That's a one-second lowering, no pause, and explosive lifting.

The ESD portion of Power 2 matches the tone of the phase, with shorter bouts of exercise with maximum effort. On the first day, we'll do a 150-yard shuttle consisting of 25 yards down and back three times, which will take roughly thirty seconds. On the second day, we'll do 60-yard ladder sprints (5, 10, and 15 yards down and back). On day three, we'll do 50-yard sprints in seven seconds.

In Power 3, we'll again do a mix of isolateral and bilateral work. Here we're taking our newfound power and elasticity and doing increased work to maximize strength and strength endurance. We'll go with a 2-0-X tempo and do the same ESD routines as in Power 1. You should beat your best times from Power 1 as well as your average times. This should show you how much you've improved in just a few weeks. That doesn't mean this becomes any easier, but you'll produce more wattage, enabling you to cover more ground in less time. ESD is about creating quality endurance. That means the longer you can hold your best time, the better shape you are in. The more you fade from the first repetition to the last, the more out of shape you are. Everyone gets tired, of course, but you want to recover quickly.

In Power 4, the movements will be similar to previous phases, but we're going to increase your stability and strength with isolateral movements and spike the intensity with bilateral movements for maximum power. The tempo here will be like Power 2 (1-0-X) so that you're using more elasticity. Your ESD will also be the same as Power 2. Again your goal is to beat both your best times and average times. Think in terms of establishing a PR (personal record) at each session, whether in terms of time (the faster the better) or amount of resistance.

The first time through the program, start off in the Foundational Power theme and then progress from Power 1 through Power 4. The Foundational phase is designed to be two weeks in length (six Power sessions) with the remaining phases to be three weeks each in length (nine Power sessions per phase). The first time through the program, it is important to adhere to that number of sessions in order to correct any dysfunctional movement patterns. At the conclusion of each Power phase, return to the Foundational phase for one-half week to allow your body to recover for your next phase. The first time through the system, your phase progression should look like this:

Week #	Phase
1–2	Foundational
3–5	Power 1
6–6.5	Foundational
6.5–8.5	Power 2
9.5–10	Foundational
10–12	Power 3
13–13.5	Foundational
13.5–15.5	Power 4
16.5–17	Foundational

As you progress through the program beyond the initial seventeen weeks, feel free to adjust the length of time in a phase to suit your goals. If, for instance, you have an important event, competition, or mission four weeks away, create a preparation cycle that consists of, say, a half week of Foundational, one week of Power 1, two weeks of Power 2, and another half week of Foundational to taper.

As you begin to mix and match phases, make it a point to insert at least half a week of Foundational every three weeks to enable your body to recover and adapt, leaving you fresh for the next phase. This program is designed to be modular and adaptable, with the phases combined in any number of ways to fit the demands and constraints of your life.

After selecting your Power phase, the next step is to determine your weekly schedule or microcycle. In the Athletes' Performance program, the microcycle is meant to be adaptable and fluid to your schedule and demands and can vary from week to week.

Each microcycle will include three Power sessions, at least one Movement Skills session, one Regeneration session, an optional complementary training ses-

Athletes' Performance Workout Equipment

You'll notice that this program requires a fair amount of equipment: dumbbells, barbell set, kettlebells, bench, blue pad, tennis ball, tennis ball "peanut," TRX Suspension Trainer, cable machine, tubing, miniband, soft tissue or foam roll, hurdles, bungee cord/belt, slides, medicine ball, jump band, massage stick, and stretch rope.

Thankfully, most of this equipment can be found in even the most bare-bones gyms. Other items you likely have already (tennis ball) or can purchase for minimal cost.

When we wrote our first book more than a decade ago, we included equipment such as med balls and foam rollers that few gyms had at the time but that now are standard.

With this program, please adopt a mindset that these tools are crucial to your success and will provide huge return on investment. Many can be packed into one compact "survival bag."

Of course, we never want to use a lack of equipment as an excuse. Many of these items travel well. And if you find yourself in a situation without equipment, there are many movements in this program you can do with no equipment using your own body weight as resistance.

Remember: A high performer finds a way to perform regardless of the environment or tools on hand.

sion (such as yoga, Pilates, cross-training, etc.), and at least one off day. Those sessions can be combined in any number of ways. Just remember that if you train four days in a row, at least one of those days needs to be a Regeneration day.

Session Type	Frequency Per Week
Power	3
Movement Skills	At least 1
Regeneration	At least 1
Complementary	Optional
Off Day	At least 1

During the Foundational phase, there are only two versions of Power sessions, and since the microcycle calls for three Power days, it takes two weeks to balance the versions, meaning you've done each version an equal number of times. During the first week, you will do the A version, then the B, and then back to A. For the second week, you will start with B, then perform the A version, and then back to B. You'll continue alternating week by week until you are ready to progress to the next phase.

Some sample microcycles for the Foundational phase:

	Monday	Tuesday	Wednesday	Thursday	Friday	Saturday	Sunday
Option A: Week 1	Power A	Movement Skills: Linear	Power B	Regeneration	Power A	Yoga	Off
Option A: Week 2	Power B	Movement Skills: Multidirectional	Power A	Regeneration	Power B	Yoga	Off
Option B: Week 1	Power A	Regeneration	Power B	Off	Power A	Movement Skills: Linear	Off
Option B: Week 2	Power B	Regeneration	Power A	Off	Power B	Movement Skills: Multidirectional	Off
Option C: Week 1	Power A	Regeneration	Power B	Movement Skills: Linear	Power A	Yoga	Off
Option C: Week 2	Power B	Regeneration	Power A	Movement Skills: Multidirectional	Power B	Yoga	Off

For all other phases, there are three Power workout variations that will be performed once per week, making the microcycle more consistent. Some sample microcycles for the remaining phases:

	Monday	Tuesday	Wednesday	Thursday	Friday	Saturday	Sunday
Option A	Power A	Movement Skills: Combination	Power B	Regeneration	Power C	Yoga	Off
Option B	Power A	Regeneration	Power B	Off	Power C	Movement Skills: Combination	Off
Option C	Power A	Movement Skills: Linear	Power B	Movement Skills: Multidirectional	Power C	Regeneration	Off

Once the microcycle is in place, the only thing you need to do is follow the appropriate workout card for that day and perform the movements listed on the prescribed version. Power A, B, and C for a particular phase can all be found on the same card. The Movement Skills sessions can be found on an individual card, as can the Regeneration sessions.

Session Layout

Within the individual training sessions there will be training components: Pillar Prep, Movement Prep, Plyometrics, Movement Skills, Medicine Ball, Relative Power, ESD, and Regeneration. These training components serve as the skeleton of a training session, providing structure throughout your workouts and ensuring you develop every aspect necessary to improve your performance.

Power Sessions

Once you select your workout card for the day of the microcycle you are on, simply follow the movements from top to bottom to complete the session. For example, look at the Strength A session for the Power 1 phase. You'll see that you have five Pillar Preparation movements followed by six Movement Preparation movements, and then two Plyometrics movements. After completing all of those movements for the prescribed number of sets and repetitions, you then move on to the Relative Power portion of the workout.

The Power workout template is designed to convey multiple weeks of loading on one sheet. Taking a close look at the template, you can see that the first block is Total Body Power, which consists of two movements: HANG SNATCH PULL and Reach, Roll, and Lift—Heel Sit (Foam Roll).

	Reverse Lunge Forearm to Instep w/Rotation	1	5 ea
	Lateral Lunge	1	5 ea
	Pillar March–Linear	2	10 steps ea
	Pillar Skip–Linear	3	10 steps ea
PL	Linear Hurdle Hop–Double Contact	2	6 ea
	Lateral Bound–Quick/Stabilize	3	6 ea

ST

	Week 1		Week 2		Week 3		eek 3
Total Body Power Block	**HANG SNATCH PULL**						
	Reach, Roll, and Lift–Heel Sit (Foam Roll) x6						
	6		5		4		
	6		5		4		
	6		5		4		
					4		

	Bent Knee Hamstring Stretch x6 ea					
	9		8		7	
	9		8		7	
	9		8		7	
					7	
	REVERSE LUNGE–DB (30x)					
	Sidelying Quad/Hip Flexor Stretch x6 ea					
	9		8		7	
	9		8		7	
	9		8		7	

There are also three columns working left to right—Week 1, Week 2, and Week 3—and working down each column, you'll see numbers of prescribed repetitions.

The numbers going vertically are always tied to the movement that is in ALL CAPS; in this case, HANG SNATCH PULL. The number to the right of the non-capitalized movement in the gray box (in this case, Reach, Roll, and Lift—Heel Sit [Foam Roll]) is the prescription for that movement.

So in this block, in the first week you would perform HANG SNATCH PULL for six repetitions followed by Reach, Roll, and Lift—Heel Sit (Foam Roll) for six reps and repeat two more times for a total of three sets. In the second week, you would perform three sets of five repetitions of HANG SNATCH PULL, and then in the third week, four sets of four repetitions.

Reverse Lunge Forearm to Instep w/Rotation	1	5 ea	
Lateral Lunge	1	5 ea	
Pillar March–Linear	2	10 steps ea	
Pillar Skip–Linear	3	10 steps ea	
PL Linear Hurdle Hop–Double Contact	2	6 ea	
Lateral Bound–Quick/Stabilize	3	6 ea	

ST

	Week 1		Week 2		Week 3		ek 3
	HANG SNATCH PULL						
	Reach, Roll, and Lift–Heel Sit (Foam Roll) x6						
Total Body Power Block	6		5		4		
	6		5		4		
	6		5		4		
					4		

	Bent Knee Hamstring Stretch x6 ea						
	9		8		7		
	9		8		7		
	9		8		7		
					7		
	REVERSE LUNGE–DB (30x)						
	Sidelying Quad/Hip Flexor Stretch x6 ea						
	9		8		7		
	9		8		7		
	9		8		7		

Working our way down the template, we start to see blocks of movements attached to each other.

This simply means that all of these movements are meant to be performed in a circuit—one right after another with no rest for the prescribed number of repetitions. In this case, during the first week, one set would be RDL (HORIZONTAL BAND, BARBELL) for nine reps, Bent-Knee Hamstring Stretch for six reps, REVERSE LUNGE (DB) for nine reps, and Sidelying Quad/Hip Flexor Stretch with Rotation for six reps. You would then repeat that circuit two more times.

To the right of the number of repetitions for the movements in ALL CAPS is a blank space for you to write down how much resistance you used for that set. Tracking your resistance will allow you to review past performances and help dial you in to your current effort to make sure you are progressing.

ST	Week 1		Week 2		Week 3	
HANG SNATCH PULL						
Reach, Roll, and Lift—Heel Sit (Foam Roll) x6						
6		5			4	

ROMANIAN DEADLIFT [RDL] (HORIZONTAL BAND, BARBELL) (30X)

Bent Knee Hamstring Stretch   x6 ea

9		8		7	
9		8		7	
9		8		7	
				7	

REVERSE LUNGE—DB (30x)

Sidelying Quad/Hip Flexor Stretch with Rotation x6 ea

9		8		7	
9		8		7	
9		8		7	
		8		7	

MOVEMENT SKILLS SESSIONS

Movement Skills templates are similar to the Power sessions, except that the loading is consistent and doesn't vary over the course of the program. There are three options to pick from: Linear, Combination, and Multidirectional. Linear days focus

MOVEMENT SKILLS—LINEAR			
Movement		Sets	Reps
PP	Foam Roll-Glutes	1	30 sec ea
	Foam Roll-IT Bands	1	30 sec ea
	Foam Roll-Quad	1	30 sec ea
	Foam Roll-Lat	14	30 sec ea
	Foam Roll-Lat	1	30 sec ea
	Foam Roll-Quad	1	30 sec ea
	Foam Roll-Lat	14	30 sec ea
	Foam Roll-Lat	1	30 sec ea
MP	Miniband Walking-Linear Bent Knee	1	5 ea
	Knee Hug	1	5 ea
	Forward Lunge w/Lateral Flexion	1	5 ea
	Drop Lunge	1	5 ea
	Pillar March-Linear	2	10 steps ea
	Pillar Skip-Linear	3	10 steps ea
	2 Inch Runs-In Place	3	6 sec
PL	Horizontal Jump-Stabilize	3	5
	Linear Bound-Quick/Stabilize	2	5 ea
MS	Wall Drill-Posture Hold	2	30 sec ea
	Wall Drill-Load and Lift	2	8 ea
	Wall Drill-Single Exchange	2	8 ea
	Sled Pull-Accelerations	3	15 yd
	Accelerations-15 yd	2	15 yd
	Sled Pull-Accelerations	3	15 yd
	Accelerations-15 yd	4	15 yd
	Sprints	2	40 yd
	Sled March-Low	4	25 yd
ESD	Your Choice	2 to 3	5:00 Hard/1:00 Easy

MOVEMENT SKILLS—COMBINATION			
Movement		Sets	Reps
PP	Foam Roll-Glutes	1	30 sec ea
	Foam Roll-IT Band	1	30 sec ea
	Foam Roll-Quad	1	30 sec ea
	Foam Roll-Lat	1	30 sec ea
	Trigger Point-Arch	1	50 ea
	Foam Roll-Quad	1	30 sec ea
	Foam Roll-Lat	1	30 sec ea
	Trigger Point-Arch	1	50 ea
MP	Miniband Walking-Linear Bent Knee	1	5 ea
	Knee Hug	1	5 ea
	Forward Lunge w/Lateral Flexion	1	5 ea
	Drop Lunge	1	5 ea
	Lateral Lunge 1	1	5 ea
	Pillar March-Linear	2	10 steps ea
	Pillar Skip-Lateral	3	10 steps ea
	2 Inch Runs-In Place	3	6 sec
PL	Horizontal Jump-Stabilize	3	5
	Linear Bound-90 deg Quick/Stabilize	2	5 ea
MS	Wall Drill-Single Exchange	2	8 ea
	Sled Pull-Accelerations	3	15 yd
	Accelerations-15 yd	2	15 yd
	Lateral Shuffle-Resisted Continuous	3	3 ea
	Lateral Shuffle-Continuous	3	3 ea
	Sprints	2	40 yd
	Sled March-Low	4	25 yd
ESD	Your Choice	2 to 3	5:00 Hard/1:00 Easy

MOVEMENT SKILLS—MULTIDIRECTIONAL			
Movement		Sets	Reps
PP	5 Way Hip Cable	1	10 ea
MP	Miniband Walking-Lateral Bent Knee	1	10 steps ea
	Lateral Lunge	1	5 ea
	Leg Cradle	1	5 ea
MP	Miniband Walking-Lateral Bent Knee	1	10 steps ea
	Lateral Lunge	1	5 ea
	Leg Cradle	1	5 ea
	Handwalk		5
	Crossover Step	2	10 steps ea
	Tinioca	2	10 steps ea
	Dropstep Skip	3	10 steps ea
	Base Rotations	3	6 sec
PL	Rotational Bound-90 deg Quick/Stabilize	3	5 ea
MS	Crossover to Base-Quick/Stabilize	2	6 ea
	Crossover to Base-Resisted Continuous	4	3 ea
	Lateral Shuffle-Resisted Quick/Stabilize	3	3 ea
	Lateral Shuffle-Quick/Stabilize	1	3 ea
	Lateral Shuffle-Resisted Continuous	3	3 ea
	Lateral Shuffle-Continuous	3	3 ea
ESD	Your Choice	2 to 3	30" Sprint/4:30 Hard/ 2 min easy
RG	Soft Tissue Routine		
	Cold Tub or Compression	1	20 min

on acceleration and absolute speed, Multidirectional days focus on crossover, shuffling, and cutting, and Combination days bring all aspects of Movement Skills into the session.

If you are doing Movement Skills sessions twice during your microcycle, go ahead and alternate between Linear and Multidirectional emphasis. If you are only doing one Movement Skills session each week, you can either choose a Combination session or alternate from week to week between Linear and Multidirectional.

Once you pick what type of session you want to do, simply work your way down the card to see what movements and loading you should do.

		MOVEMENT SKILLS—LINEAR			
PP	Foam Roll–Glutes		1	30 sec ea	**Reps**
	Foam Roll–IT Bands		1	30 sec ea	30 sec ea
	Foam Roll–Quad		1	30 sec ea	30 sec ea
	Foam Roll–Lat		14	30 sec ea	30 sec ea
	Foam Roll–Lat		1	30 sec ea	30 sec ea
					30 sec ea
	MP	Miniband Walking–Linear Bent Knee	1	5 ea	
		Knee Hug	1	5 ea	
		Forward Lunge w/Lateral Flexion	1	5 ea	
		Drop Lunge	1	5 ea	
		Pillar March–Linear	2	10 steps ea	
		Pillar Skip–Linear	3	10 steps ea	
		2 Inch Runs–In Place	3	6 sec	
	PL	Horizontal Jump–Stabilize	3	5	
		Linear Bound–Quick/Stabilize	2	5 ea	
	MS	Wall Drill–Posture Hold	2	30 sec ea	
		Wall Drill–Load and Lift	2	8 ea	
		Wall Drill–Single Exchange	2	8 ea	
		Sled Pull–Accelerations	3	15 yd	
		Accelerations–15 yd	2	15 yd	
		Sled Pull–Accelerations	3	15 yd	
		Accelerations–15 yd	4	15 yd	
		Sprints	2	40 yd	
		Sled March–Low	4	25 yd	
	ESD	Your Choice	2 to 3	5:00 Hard/1:00 Easy	
	RG	Soft Tissue Routine			
		Cold Tub or Compression			

ENERGY SYSTEMS DEVELOPMENT SESSIONS

You will find the ESD portion at the end of each Power and Movement Skills session, as we develop programs from quality to quality endurance. Imagine a pyramid with quality at the top and working down toward quality endurance near the bottom, and now impose this over this workout, and you figuratively understand the science behind quality training. Each session begins with quality and leads to quality endurance toward the end.

You'll see ESD, then a series of sets in the first column, then the reps, distance, and rest intervals in the next column. Make sure to have a timing device and your relentless determination ready to produce and sustain some wattage. Remember, everyone gets tired; you are aiming to produce the highest amount of wattage during the sessions and recover faster and more completely between reps, sets, and days. Your newly found and mastered breathing skills will serve you well in elevating your performance.

REGENERATION SESSIONS

There are seven options of Regeneration sessions to pick from: General Regeneration, Self-Massage, Flexibility, Upper Back/Shoulder Pain, Low Back Pain, Hip Pain, and Knee Pain. Wherever your Regeneration session falls during the microcycle, simply pick which type of session you want to do and follow those movements on the card. In addition to having Regeneration sessions, you can also do any of the movements at the end of a Power or Movement Skills session.

COMPLEMENTARY SESSIONS

In addition to the Power, Movement Skills, and Regeneration sessions, you should feel free to schedule in at least one day of some other fun activity. Yoga and Pilates sessions are fantastic for balancing your body in a lower-impact fashion. Often we neglect to give our bodies the mobility and stability they need, and these types of classes are a great way to build in those qualities organically.

Other activities such as swimming, hiking, rock climbing, cycling, etc., are fun and effective ways to keep your week fresh. You also can see tangible performance gains related to each, which will help keep you motivated.

GENERAL REGENERATION		
Movement	**Sets**	**Reps**
ESD Your Choice	1	20 min Easy
RG Trigger Point—Thoracic Spine	1	5 ea
Trigger Point—Glutes	4	45 sec ea
Trigger Point—TFL	1	45 sec ea
Trigger Point—Neck	1	45 sec
Foam Roll—Upper Back	1	45 sec
Foam Roll—Low Back	1	45 sec ea
Foam Roll—Glutes	1	45 sec ea
Foam Roll—IT Band	1	45 sec ea
Foam Roll—Quadriceps	1	45 sec ea
Reach, Roll, and Lift—Heel Sit (Foam Roll)	1	10
Bent Knee Hamstring Stretch	1	10 ea
Abductor Stretch—Rope	1	10 ea

FLEXIBILITY		
Movement	**Sets**	**Reps**
ESD Your Choice	1	20 min Easy
RG Trigger Point—Arch/Plantar Fascia	2	50 ea
Reach, Roll, and Lift—Heel Sit (Foam Roll)	2	10
Bent Knee Hamstring Stretch	2	10 ea
Abductor Stretch—Supine (Rope)	2	10 ea
Supine Hip Internal Rotation Stretch	2	10 ea
Quad Hip Flexor Stretch—1/2 Kneeling	2	10 ea
90—90 Stretch with Arm Sweep	2	10 ea
Sidelying Shoulder Stretch	2	10 ea
Quad/Hip Flexor Stretch—Sidelying	2	10 ea

LOW BACK PAIN		
Movement	**Sets**	**Reps**
ESD Your Choice	1	20 min Easy
RG Trigger Point—Thoracic Spine	1	5 ea
Massage Stick—Low Back	1	45 sec
Trigger Point—Glutes	1	45 sec ea
Trigger Point—TFL	1	45 sec ea
Foam Roll—Thoracic Spine	2	45 sec
Foam Roll—Low Back	2	45 sec ea
Foam Roll—Glutes	2	45 sec ea
Foam Roll—Hamstrings	2	45 sec ea
Foam Roll—Quadriceps	2	45 sec ea
Reach, Roll, and Lift—Heel Sit (Foam Roll)	2	10
Bent Knee Hamstring Stretch	2	10 ea
Quad/Hip Flexor Stretch—Half Kneeling	2	10 ea
90-90 Stretch with Arm Sweep	2	10 ea

KNEE PAIN		
Movement	**Sets**	**Reps**
ESD Your Choice	1	20 min Easy
RG Massage Stick—Quadriceps	1	45 sec ea
Massage Stick—Hamstrings	1	45 sec ea
Massage Stick—TFL	1	45 sec ea
Trigger Point—Glutes	1	45 sec ea
Trigger Point—VMO	1	10 ea
Trigger Point—TFL	1	45 sec ea
Foam Roll—Glutes	2	45 sec ea
Foam Roll—Hamstrings	2	45 sec ea
Foam Roll—IT Band	2	45 sec ea
Foam Roll—Quadriceps	2	45 sec ea
Foam Roll—Adductor	2	45 sec ea
Foam Roll—Tibialis Anterior	2	45 sec

SELF MASSAGE		
Movement	**Sets**	**Reps**
ESD Your Choice	1	20 min Easy
RG Trigger Point—Thoracic Spine	1	5 ea
Trigger Point—Glutes	4	45 sec ea
Trigger Point—TFL	1	45 sec ea
Trigger Point—VMO	2	10 ea
Trigger Point—Arch/Plantar Fascia	1	50 ea
Trigger Point—Neck	1	45 sec
Foam Roll—Thoracic Spine	1	45 sec
Foam Roll—Low Back	1	45 sec ea
Foam Roll—Glutes	1	45 sec ea
Foam Roll—Hamstrings	1	45 sec ea
Foam Roll—Calf	1	45 sec ea
Foam Roll—Quadriceps	1	45 sec ea
Foam Roll—Adductor	1	45 sec ea

UPPER BACK/SHOULDER PAIN		
Movement	**Sets**	**Reps**
ESD Your Choice	1	20 min Easy
RG Massage Stick—Neck	1	45 sec
Trigger Point—Thoracic Spine	1	5 ea
Trigger Point—Neck	1	45 sec
Foam Roll—Thoracic Spine	2	45 sec
Foam Roll—Low Back	2	45 sec ea
Foam Roll—Latissimus Dorsi	2	45 sec ea
Foam Roll—Chest	2	45 sec ea
Reach, Roll, and Lift—Heel Sit (Foam Roll)	2	10
Sidelying Shoulder Stretch	2	10 ea

HIP PAIN		
Movement	**Sets**	**Reps**
ESD Your Choice	1	20 min Easy
RG Massage Stick—TFL	1	45 sec ea
Trigger Point—Glutes	1	45 sec ea
Foam Roll—Glutes	2	45 sec ea
Foam Roll—Hamstrings	2	45 sec ea
Foam Roll—IT Band	2	45 sec ea
Foam Roll—Quadriceps	2	45 sec ea
Bent Knee Hamstring Stretch	2	10 ea
Abductor Stretch—Rope	2	10 ea
Supine Hip Internal Rotation Stretch	2	10 ea
Quad/Hip Flexor Stretch—Half Kneeling	2	10 ea

SESSION TEMPLATES

Foundational

POWER A

	Movement	Sets	Reps
PP	Foam Roll—Glute	1	30 sec ea
	Foam Roll—IT Band	1	30 sec ea
	Foam Roll—Quadriceps	1	30 sec ea
	Foam Roll—Latissimus Dorsi	1	30 sec ea
	Trigger Point—Arch/Plantar Fascia	1	50 sec
MP	Inverted Hamstring	1	5 ea
	Knee Hug	1	5 ea
	Reverse Lunge—Forearm to Instep with Rotation	1	5 ea
	Lateral Lunge	1	5 ea
	Pillar March—Linear	2	10 steps ea
	Pillar Skip—Linear	3	10 steps ea
PL	Drop Squat—2 Foot to 1 Foot	2	6 ea
	Linear Hurdle Hop—Countermovement	2	6 ea
	Lateral Bound—Stabilize (Miniband)	3	6 ea

Total Body Power Block

RP	Session 1	Session 3	Session 5	
OVERHEAD ROTATIONAL SQUAT—1 ARM KB				
Deep Squat to Hamstring Stretch			x6	
Lateral Pillar Bridge to Row—w/Hip Flexion			x6	
9 ea	8 ea	7 ea		
9 ea	8 ea	7 ea		

Primary & Secondary Block

BENCH PRESS—ALT DB w/ LEG LOWERING (21x)				
Sliding Overhead Press			x6	
8 ea	9 ea	10 ea		
8 ea	9 ea	10 ea		
8 ea	9 ea	10 ea		

RDL TO ROW—1 ARM, 1 LEG (CABLE) (21x)				
Inverted Hamstring w/Rotation			x6 ea	
8 ea	9 ea	10 ea		
8 ea	9 ea	10 ea		
8 ea	9 ea	10 ea		

PULL UP—3 POINT ISOMETRIC HOLDS				
Trigger Point—Thoracic Spine			x5 ea	
10 sec ea	15 sec ea	20 sec ea		
10 sec ea	15 sec ea	20 sec ea		
10 sec ea	15 sec ea	20 sec ea		

SPLIT SQUAT—1 ARM DB (21x)				
Quad Hip Flexor Stretch—Half Kneeling			x6 ea	
8 ea	9 ea	10 ea		
8 ea	9 ea	10 ea		
8 ea	9 ea	10 ea		

Rotational Block

STABILITY CHOP—HALF KNEELING (CABLE)				
Dynamic Pillar Bridge (TRX)			x10 ea	
8 ea	9 ea	10 ea		
8 ea	9 ea	10 ea		

SHOULDER PRESS—w/LATERAL FLEXION (KB)				
8 ea	9 ea	10 ea		
8 ea	9 ea	10 ea		

ESD	ESD MACHINE 30 SEC HARD/4:30 MIN MODERATE				
	1		2	1 min rest	3	1 min rest

RG Soft Tissue Routine
Cold Tub/Compression Boots

POWER B

	Movement	Sets	Reps
PP	5-Way Hip Cable	1	10 ea
MP	Leg Cradle	1	5 ea
	Dropstep Squat	1	5 ea
	Drop Lunge	1	5 ea
	Handwalk	1	5
	Pillar March—Lateral	2	10 steps ea
	Lateral Pillar Skip—Lateral	3	10 steps ea
MB	Chest Pass—1 Leg	2	10 ea
	Overhead Pass—1 Leg	2	10 ea
	Parallel Rotational Throw—Kneeling	2	10 ea
	Perpendicular Rotational Throw—1 Leg	2	10 ea

RP	Session 2	Session 4	Session 6	
OVERHEAD SQUAT—SLIDES				
Turkish Get Up (KB)			x3ea	
9	8	7		
9	8	7		

BENT-OVER ROW—1 ARM 1 LEG IPSILATERAL (DB) (21x)				
Inverted Hamstring w/Rotation			x6 ea	
8 ea	9 ea	10 ea		
8 ea	9 ea	10 ea		
8 ea	9 ea	10 ea		

LEG CURL—ECCENTRIC (SLIDE) (51x)				
Quad/Hip Flexor Stretch—Half Kneeling			x6 ea	
4	5	6		
4	5	6		
4	5	6		

REVERSE LUNGE TO ROW (21x)				
Reach, Roll, and Lift—Heel Sit (Foam Roll)			x6 ea	
10 ea	9 ea	8 ea		
10 ea	9 ea	8 ea		
10 ea	9 ea	8 ea		

LATERAL LUNGE—CONTALATERAL BOTTOM-UP KB (SLIDE) (21x)				
Quadruped Rocking (Wide)			x6	
8 ea	9 ea	10 ea		
8 ea	9 ea	10 ea		
8 ea	9 ea	10 ea		

STABILITY LIFT—HALF KNEELING (CABLE)				
Pillar Bridge—Row to Tricep Extension			x10 ea	
8 ea	9 ea	10 ea		
8 ea	9 ea	10 ea		

ESD	ESD MACHINE 1:00 MIN HARD/1:00 MIN EASY				
	2 x 4	2 min rest	2 x 5	2 min rest	2 x 6	2 min rest

RG Soft Tissue Routine
Cold Tub/Compression Boots

Power 1

POWER A

	Movement	Sets	Reps
PP	Toe Finger Weave—Circles	1	10 ea
	Hip Internal Rotation—Sidelying with Abduction	1	10 ea
	Segmental Glute Bridge	1	10 ea
	Lateral Line Stretch—Standing	2	4x3 Breaths ea
	Quad Thoracic Spine Rotation—1 Leg Abduction	1	4 ea
MP	Inverted Hamstring	1	5 ea
	Knee Hug	1	5 ea
	Reverse Lunge Forearm to Instep w/Rotation	1	5 ea
	Lateral Lunge	1	5 ea
	Pillar March—Linear	2	10 steps ea
	Pillar Skip—Linear	3	10 steps ea
PL	Linear Hurdle Hop—Double Contact	3	6 ea
	Lateral Bound—Quick and Stabilize	3	6 ea

POWER A — RP (Total Body Power Block)

RP	Week 1	Week 2	Week 3
	HANG SNATCH PULL		
	Reach, Roll, and Lift—Heel Sit (Foam Roll)		x6
	6	5	4
	6	5	4
	6	5	4
			4

Primary & Secondary Block

	Week 1	Week 2	Week 3
	ROMANIAN DEADLIFT [RDL] (HORIZONTAL BAND, BARBELL) (30x)		
	Bent Knee Hamstring Stretch		x6 ea
	9	8	7
	9	8	7
	9	8	7
		8	7
	REVERSE LUNGE—DB (30x)		
	Sidelying Quad/Hip Flexor Stretch with Rotation		x6 ea
	9	8	7
	9	8	7
	9	8	7
		8	7

Rotational Block

	Week 1	Week 2	Week 3
	ROTATIONAL ROW (21x)		
	Adductor Stretch—Half Kneeling		x6 ea
	8 ea	7 ea	6 ea
	8 ea	7 ea	6 ea

Auxiliary Block

	Week 1	Week 2	Week 3
	LEG CURL—1 LEG (STABILITY BALL)		
	8 ea	10 ea	12 ea
	8 ea	10 ea	12 ea
	LATERAL PILLAR BRIDGE TO ROW (w/ HIP FLEXION)		
	12 ea	10 ea	8 ea
	12 ea	10 ea	8 ea
	LATERAL LUNGE—CONTRALATERAL BOTTOM UP KB (SLIDE)		
	12 ea	10 ea	8 ea
	12 ea	10 ea	8 ea
	PILLAR BRIDGE TO ROW TO TRICEP EXTENSION (CABLE)		
	12 ea	10 ea	8 ea
	12 ea	10 ea	8 ea

ESD	**300-YARD SHUTTLE**					
	4	3 min rest	5	3 min rest	6	3 min rest

RG Soft Tissue Routine
Cold Tub/Compression Boots

POWER B

	Movement	Sets	Reps
PP	Toe Wall Walks	1	6
	Prone Breathing Over Physioball	2	5 Breaths
	Hip Internal Rotation—Sidelying with Abduction	1	10 ea
	Sidelying Quad/Hip Flexor Stretch with Rotation	2	4x3 Breaths ea
	Quad Thoracic Spine Rotation w/Rot with 1 Leg Ext	1	4 ea
MP	Leg Cradle	1	5 ea
	Dropstep Squat	1	5 ea
	Drop Lunge	1	5 ea
	Handwalk	1	5
	Pillar March—Lateral	2	10 steps ea
	Pillar Skip—Lateral	3	10 steps ea
PL	Chest Pass—Split Squat	2	10 ea
	Overhead Pass—Split Squat	2	10 ea
	Parallel Rotational Throw—Split Squat	2	10 ea

POWER B — RP

RP	Week 1	Week 2	Week 3
	SQUAT TO PRESS THROW		
	Quadruped Rocking		x6
	6	5	4
	6	5	4
	6	5	4

	Week 1	Week 2	Week 3
	PULL-UP (30x)		
	Reach, Roll, and Lift—Heel Sit Foam Roll)		x6
	9	8	7
	9	8	7
	9	8	7
		8	7
	BENCH PRESS—ALT DB WITH LEG LOWERING (30x)		
	Sliding Overhead Press—Floor		x6
	9	8	7
	9	8	7
	9	8	7
		8	7

	Week 1	Week 2	Week 3
	CABLE CHOP—LATERAL, HALF KNEELING (21x)		
	Supine Hip Rotator Stretch		x6
	8 ea	7 ea	6 ea
	8 ea	7 ea	6 ea

	Week 1	Week 2	Week 3
	PULLOVER EXTENSION—ALT DB WITH HIP EXTENSION		
	12	10	8
	12	10	8
	DYNAMIC PILLAR BRIDGE (TRX)		
	8	10	12
	8	10	12
	SHOULDER PRESS WITH LATERAL FLEXION (KB)		
	12 ea	10 ea	8 ea
	12 ea	10 ea	8 ea
	90-90 STRETCH WITH ARM SWEEP		
	6 ea	6 ea	6 ea
	6 ea	6 ea	6 ea

ESD	**LADDER SHUTTLE DRILL (5-10-15-20-25)**					
	2x3	2 min rest	2x4	90 sec rest	2x5	1 min rest

RG Soft Tissue Routine
Cold Tub/Compression Boots

POWER C

	Movement	Sets	Reps
PP	Inverted Hamstring	1	5 ea
	Leg Cradle	1	5 ea
	Knee Hug	1	5 ea
	Lateral Lunge	1	5 ea
	Reverse Lunge—Forearm to Instep with Rotation	1	5 ea
	Dropstep Skip	3	10 steps ea
PL	Lateral Hurdle Hop—Double Contact	2	6 ea
	Squat Jump—Non-countermovement	3	4
MB	Walking Lunge to Chest Pass—NCM	2	5 ea
	Parallel Rotational Throw—Standing	2	10 ea
	Perpendicular Rotational Throw—Standing	2	10 ea

POWER C — RP

RP	Week 1	Week 2	Week 3

	Week 1	Week 2	Week 3
	BENT-OVER ROW—1 ARM 1 LEG (DB—CONTRALATERAL) (30x)		
	Foam Roll—Lat		x20 sec ea
	10	9	8
	10	9	8
	10	9	8
	SQUAT—1 LEG FRONT LOADED (DB) (30x)		
	Foam Roll—Quadriceps		x20 sec ea
	10	9	8
	10	9	8
	10	9	8
	BENCH PRESS—1 ARM, OFF BENCH (30x)		
	Foam Roll—Pec		x20 sec ea
	10	9	8
	10	9	8
	10	9	8
	RDL—2 ARM 1 LEG DB (30x)		
	Foam Roll—Glute		x20 sec ea
	10	9	8
	10	9	8
	10	9	8

	Week 1	Week 2	Week 3
	ROTATIONAL PUSH/PULL (21x)		
	90—90 Stretch w/Arm Sweep		x6 ea
	8 ea	7 ea	6 ea
	8 ea	7 ea	6 ea

	Week 1	Week 2	Week 3
	PUSH-UP		
	30 sec	35 sec	40 sec
	30 sec	35 sec	40 sec
	LEG CURL—ECCENTRIC (SLIDE)		
	30 sec	35 sec	40 sec
	30 sec	35 sec	40 sec
	PULLDOWN—ALTERNATING		
	30 sec	35 sec	40 sec
	30 sec	35 sec	40 sec
	SQUAT TO PRESS—1 ARM (DB)		
	30 sec	35 sec	40 sec
	30 sec	35 sec	40 sec

ESD	**100 YD SPRINTS**					
	6	1 min rest	8	1 min rest	10	1 min rest

RG Soft Tissue Routine
Cold Tub/Compression Boots

Power 2

POWER A

	Movement	Sets	Reps
PP	Toe Waves	2	5 ea
	Segmental Glute Bridge with Lateral Shift	2	6 ea
	Quad/Hip Flexor Stretch—Half Kneel with Lateral Flex	2	4x3 Breaths Ea
	Quadruped Weight Shifts	2	4 ea
	Supine Active Hip Rotator Stretch	2	10 ea
MP	Inverted Hamstring	1	5 ea
	Knee Hug	1	5 ea
	Reverse Lunge Forearm to Instep with Rotation	1	5 ea
	Lateral Lunge	1	5 ea
	Pillar March—Linear	2	10 steps ea
	Pillar Skip—Linear	3	10 steps ea
PL	Linear Hurdle Hop—Continuous	2	6 ea
	Lateral Bound—Continuous	3	6 ea

RP	Week 1	Week 2	Week 3

HANG SNATCH—1 ARM (DB)

Reach, Roll, and Lift—Heel Sit (Foam Roll)		x6	
5 ea	4 ea	3 ea	
5 ea	4 ea	3 ea	
5 ea	4 ea	3 ea	

Total Body Power Block

SPLIT SQUAT—BACK FOOT ELEVATED (DB) (10x)

*Split Squat Jump—BACK FOOT ELEVATED		x4 ea	
Quad/Hip Flexor Stretch—Sidelying		x6 ea	
7 ea	6 ea*	5 ea*	
6 ea*	5 ea*	4 ea*	
6 ea*	5 ea*	4 ea*	
6 ea*	5 ea*	4 ea*	

RDL—2 ARM, 1 LEG (DB) (10x)

*Straight-Leg Skip		x6 steps ea	
Bent-Knee Hamstring Stretch		x6 ea	
7 ea	6 ea	5 ea	
6 ea*	5 ea*	4 ea*	
6 ea*	5 ea*	4 ea*	
6 ea*	5 ea*	4 ea*	

Primary & Secondary Block

ROTATIONAL ROW—REACTIVE (xxx)

Adductor Stretch—Half Kneeling		x6 ea	
6 ea	5 ea	4 ea	
6 ea	5 ea	4 ea	

Rotational Block

LATERAL LUNGE—HORIZONTAL RESISTANCE (SLIDE)

10 ea	8 ea	6 ea	
10 ea	8 ea	6 ea	

LATERAL PILLAR BRIDGE TO ROW—WITH HIP FLEXION

8 ea	10 ea	12 ea	
8 ea	10 ea	12 ea	

REVERSE LUNGE—HORIZONTAL RESISTANCE (SLIDE)

10 ea	8 ea	6 ea	
10 ea	8 ea	6 ea	

PILLAR BRIDGE—DYNAMIC ALTERNATING (ARMS IN TRX)

8 ea	10 ea	12 ea	
8 ea	10 ea	12 ea	

Auxiliary Block

ESD — 150- YARD SHUTTLE

2x4	60 sec rest	2x5	45 sec rest	2x6	30 sec rest

RG Soft Tissue Routine
Cold Tub/Compression Boots

POWER B

	Movement	Sets	Reps
PP	Standing Toe Taps	2	5 ea
	Step to Inverted Hamstring Stretch	2	6 ea
	Sidelying Quad/Hip Flexor Stretch with Rotation	2	4x3 Breaths Ea
	Supine Fallout at 90 Hip Flexion with FL Connect	2	6 ea
	Fencing Stretch	2	8 ea
MP	Leg Cradle	1	5 ea
	Dropstep Squat	1	5 ea
	Drop Lunge	1	5 ea
	Handwalk	1	5
	Pillar March—Lateral	2	10 steps ea
	Pillar Skip—Lateral	3	10 steps ea
PL	Chest Pass—Standing	3	10
	Overhead Throw	3	5 ea
	Perpendicular Rotational Throw—Standing	3	10 ea

RP	Week 1	Week 2	Week 3

BOX JUMP

Quadruped Rocking		x6	
4	5	6	
4	5	6	
4	5	6	

PULL-UP (10x)

*Overhead Slam (MB)		x4	
Reach, Roll, and Lift—Heel Sit (Foam Roll)		x6	
7	6	5	
6*	5*	4*	
6*	5*	4*	
6*	5*	4*	

BENCH PRESS—1 ARM (DB) (10x)

*Push-Up On Bench—Countermovement (Plyo)		x4	
Sliding Overhead Press		x6	
7 ea	6 ea	5 ea	
6 ea*	5 ea*	4 ea*	
6 ea*	5 ea*	4 ea*	
6 ea*	5 ea*	4 ea*	

ROTATIONAL CHOP—STANDING (10x)

Supine Hip Rotator Stretch		x6	
6 ea	5 ea	4 ea	
6 ea	5 ea	4 ea	

ROTATIONAL ROW (TRX)

10 ea	8 ea	6 ea	
10 ea	8 ea	6 ea	

PRONE KNEE TUCK (TRX)

8	10	12	
8	10	12	

PUSH UP (TRX)

10	8	6	
10	8	6	

90-90 STRETCH WITH ARM SWEEP

6 ea	6 ea	6 ea	
6 ea	6 ea	6 ea	

ESD — LADDER SHUTTLE DRILL (5-10-15)

2x4	60 sec rest	2x5	45 sec rest	2x6	30 sec rest

RG Soft Tissue Routine
Cold Tub/Compression Boots

POWER C

	Movement	Sets	Reps
PP	Inverted Hamstring	1	5 ea
	Leg Cradle	1	5 ea
	Knee Hug	1	5 ea
	Lateral Lunge	1	5 ea
	Reverse Lunge—Forearm to Instep with Rotation	1	5 ea
	Dropstep Skip	3	10 steps ea
PL	Lateral Hurdle Hop—Continuous	3	6 ea
	Squat Jump—Countermovement	3	4
MB	Walking Lunge to Chest Pass	2	5 ea
	Parallel Rotational Throw—Standing	2	10 ea
	Perpendicular Rotational Throw—Standing	2	10 ea
	Granny Toss	3	5

RP	Week 1	Week 2	Week 3

BENT-OVER ROW—1 ARM (DB) (10x)

Foam Roll—Latissimus Dorsi		x20 sec ea	
7 ea	6 ea	5 ea	
7 ea	6 ea	5 ea	
7 ea	6 ea	5 ea	

FRONT SQUAT—(BARBELL) (10x)

Foam Roll—Quadriceps		x20 sec ea	
7	6	5	
7	6	5	
7	6	5	

BENCH PRESS (DB) (10x)

Foam Roll—Chest		x20 sec ea	
7	6	5	
7	6	5	
7	6	5	

RDL (BARBELL) (10x)

Foam Roll—Glute		x20 sec ea	
7	6	5	
7	6	5	
7	6	5	

ROTATIONAL PUSH/PULL—REACTIVE (xxx)

90—90 Stretch with Arm Sweep		x6 ea	
6 ea	5 ea	4 ea	
6 ea	5 ea	4 ea	

PULLDOWN—ALTERNATING

12 ea	10 ea	8 ea	
12 ea	10 ea	8 ea	

REVERSE LUNGE—ALTERNATING (DB)

12 ea	10 ea	8 ea	
12 ea	10 ea	8 ea	

INCLINE BENCH PRESS—ALTERNATING (DB)

12 ea	10 ea	8 ea	
12 ea	10 ea	8 ea	

LEG CURL (SLIDE)

8	10	12	
8	10	12	

ESD — 50 YD SPRINTS

2x6	30 sec rest	2x8	30 sec rest	2x10	30 sec rest

RG Soft Tissue Routine
Cold Tub/Compression Boots

Power 3

POWER A

	Movement	Sets	Reps
PP	Toe Finger Weave—Circles	1	10 ea
	Hip Internal Rotation—Sidelying with Abduction	2	10 ea
	Segmental Glute Bridge	2	10 ea
	Lateral Line Stretch—Standing	2	4x3 Breaths ea
	Quad Thoracic Spine Rotation—1 Leg Abduction	1	4 ea
MP	Inverted Hamstring	1	5 ea
	Knee Hug	1	5 ea
	Reverse Lunge—Forearm to Instep with Rotation	1	5 ea
	Lateral Lunge	1	5 ea
	Pillar March—Linear	2	10 steps ea
	Pillar Skip—Linear	3	10 steps ea
PL	Linear Hurdle Hop—Double Contact (Weight Vest)	2	6 ea
	Lateral Bound—Quick and Stabilize (Weight Vest)	2	6 ea

RP	Week 1	Week 2	Week 3

Total Body Power Block

HANG SNATCH PULL

Reach, Roll, and Lift—Heel Sit (Foam Roll)   x6

Week 1	Week 2	Week 3	
6	5	4	
6	5	4	
6	5	4	

Primary & Secondary Block

REVERSE LUNGE (DB) (20x)

Quad/Hip Flexor Stretch—Half Kneeling   x6 ea

Week 1	Week 2	Week 3	
8 ea	7 ea	6 ea	
8 ea	7 ea	6 ea	
7 ea	6 ea	5 ea	
7 ea	6 ea	5 ea	

RDL—2 ARM, 1 LEG (DB) (20x)

Straight Leg Lowering   x6 ea

Week 1	Week 2	Week 3	
8 ea	7 ea	6 ea	
8 ea	7 ea	6 ea	
7 ea	6 ea	5 ea	
7 ea	6 ea	5 ea	

Rotational Block

ROTATIONAL LIFT (11x)

Adductor Stretch—Half Kneeling   x6 ea

Week 1	Week 2	Week 3	
8 ea	7 ea	6 ea	
8 ea	7 ea	6 ea	

Auxiliary Block

LEG CURL—1 LEG (STABILITY BALL)

8 ea	10 ea	12 ea	
8 ea	10 ea	12 ea	

LATERAL PILLAR BRIDGE TO ROW WITH HIP FLEXION

10 ea	8 ea	6 ea	
10 ea	8 ea	6 ea	

LATERAL LUNGE—CONTRALATERAL BOTTOM-UP KB (SLIDE)

10 ea	8 ea	6 ea	
10 ea	8 ea	6 ea	

PILLAR BRIDGE—ROW TO TRICEP EXTENSION

10 ea	8 ea	6 ea	
10 ea	8 ea	6 ea	

ESD — 300-YD SHUTTLES

6	2 min rest	7	90 sec rest	8	1 min rest

RG   Soft Tissue Routine
Cold Tub/Compression Boots

POWER B

	Movement	Sets	Reps
PP	Toe Wall Walks	1	6
	Prone Breathing Over Stability Ball	2	5 breaths
	Hip Internal Rotation—Sidelying with Abduction	2	10 ea
	Sidelying Quad/Hip Flexor Stretch w/Rotation	2	4x3 breaths ea
	Quad Thoracic Spine Rotation—1 Leg Extended Ext	1	4 ea
MP	Leg Cradle	1	5 ea
	Dropstep Squat	1	5 ea
	Drop Lunge	1	5 ea
	Handwalk	1	5
	Pillar March—Lateral	2	10 steps ea
	Pillar Skip—Lateral	3	10 steps ea
MB	Chest Pass—Split Squat	2	10 ea
	Overhead Pass—Split Squat	2	10 ea
	Parallel Rotational Throw—Split Squat	3	10 ea

RP	Week 1	Week 2	Week 3

PUSH PRESS

Quadruped Rocking   x6

Week 1	Week 2	Week 3	
6	5	4	
6	5	4	
6	5	4	

BENT OVER ROW—1 ARM 1 LEG (DB—CONTRALATERAL) (20x)

Inverted Hamstring with Rotation   x6 ea

Week 1	Week 2	Week 3	
8 ea	7 ea	6 ea	
8 ea	7 ea	6 ea	
7 ea	6 ea	5 ea	
7 ea	6 ea	5 ea	

BENCH PRESS—ALT DB w/LEG LOWERING (ANKLE WEIGHTS) (20x)

Sliding Overhead Press   x6

Week 1	Week 2	Week 3	
8 ea	7 ea	6 ea	
8 ea	7 ea	6 ea	
7 ea	6 ea	5 ea	
7 ea	6 ea	5 ea	

CABLE CHOP—LATERAL HALF KNEELING (11x)

Supine Hip Rotator Stretch   x6

Week 1	Week 2	Week 3	
8 ea	7 ea	6 ea	
8 ea	7 ea	6 ea	

PULLOVER EXTENSION—DB WITH ALT HIP EXTENSION

10 ea	8 ea	6 ea	
10 ea	8 ea	6 ea	

PILLAR BRIDGE—DYNAMIC ALTERNATING (TRX)

8 ea	10 ea	12 ea	
8 ea	10 ea	12 ea	

SHOULDER PRESS WITH LATERAL FLEXION (KB)

10 ea	8 ea	6 ea	
10 ea	8 ea	6 ea	

90-90 STRETCH WITH ARM SWEEP

6 ea	8 ea	6 ea	
6 ea	8 ea	6 ea	

ESD — LADDER SHUTTLE DRILL (5-10-15-20-25)

2x6	2 min rest	2x7	90 sec rest	2x8	1 min rest

RG   Soft Tissue Routine
Cold Tub/Compression Boots

POWER C

	Movement	Sets	Reps
PP	Inverted Hamstring	1	5 ea
	Leg Cradle	1	5 ea
	Knee Hug	1	5 ea
	Lateral Lunge	1	5 ea
	Reverse Lunge Forearm to Instep w/Rotation	1	5 ea
	Dropstep Skip	3	10 steps ea
PL	Lateral Hurdle Hop—Double Contact to Stab (Weight Vest)	2	6 ea
	Squat Jump—NCM	2	4
MB	Walking Lunge to Chest Pass—NCM	2	5 ea
	Parallel Rotational Throw—Standing	2	10 ea
	Perpendicular Rotational Throw—1 Leg	3	10 ea

RP	Week 1	Week 2	Week 3

PULL-UP (20x)

Foam Roll–Latissimus Dorsi   x20 sec ea

Week 1	Week 2	Week 3	
9	8	7	
9	8	7	
9	8	7	

KETTLEBELL SWING (xxx)

Foam Roll—Glutes   x20 sec ea

Week 1	Week 2	Week 3	
9	8	7	
9	8	7	
9	8	7	

BENCH PRESS (DB) (20x)

Foam Roll—Pec   x20 sec ea

9	8	7	
9	8	7	
9	8	7	

LEG CURL (SLIDE) (20x)

Foam Roll—Hamstrings   x20 sec ea

9	8	7	
9	8	7	
9	8	7	

ROTATIONAL PUSH/PULL (11x)

90-90 Stretch with Arm Sweep   x6 ea

8 ea	7 ea	6 ea	
8 ea	7 ea	6 ea	

PUSH-UP

30 sec	35 sec	40 sec	
30 sec	35 sec	40 sec	

RDL (DB)

30 sec	35 sec	40 sec	
30 sec	35 sec	40 sec	

PULLDOWN—ALTERNATING

30 sec	35 sec	40 sec	
30 sec	35 sec	40 sec	

SQUAT TO PRESS—1 ARM (DB)

30 sec	35 sec	40 sec	
30 sec	35 sec	40 sec	

ESD — 100-YD SPRINTS

6	1 min rest	8	1 min rest	10	1 min rest

RG   Soft Tissue Routine
Cold Tub/Compression Boots

Power 4

POWER A

	Movement	Sets	Reps
PP	Toe Waves	2	5 ea
	Segmental Glute Bridge w/Lateral Shift	2	6 ea
	Quad/Hip Flexor Stretch—Half Kneel w/Lateral Fix	2	4x3 breaths ea
	Quadruped Weight Shift	2	4 ea
	Supine Active Hip Rotator Stretch	2	10 ea
MP	Inverted Hamstring	1	5 ea
	Knee Hug	1	5 ea
	Reverse Lunge—Forearm to Instep w/Rotation	1	5 ea
	Lateral Lunge	1	5 ea
	Pillar March—Linear	2	10 steps ea
	Pillar Skip—Linear	3	10 steps ea
PL	Linear Hurdle Hop—Continuous (Weight Vest)	3	6 ea
	Lateral Bound—Quick and Stabilize (Weight Vest)	3	6 ea

RP	Week 1	Week 2	Week 3
	HANG SNATCH		
	Reach, Roll, and Lift—Heel Sit (Foam Roll)		x6
	5	4	3
	5	4	3
	5	4	3

	Week 1	Week 2	Week 3
	FRONT SQUAT (BARBELL) (10x)		
	*Squat Jump		x6
	Quad/Hip Flexor Stretch—sidelying		x6 ea
	6	5	4
	5*	4*	3*
	5*	4*	3*
	5*	4*	3*
	ROMANIAN DEADLIFT (RDL) (VERTICAL BAND, BARBELL) (10x)		
	*Straight Leg Skip		x6 steps ea
	Straight Leg Lowering		x6
	6	5	4
	5*	4*	3*
	5*	4*	3*
	5*	4*	3*

	Week 1	Week 2	Week 3
	ROTATIONAL LIFT—REACTIVE (xxx)		
	Adductor Stretch—Half Kneeling		x6 ea
	6 ea	5 ea	4 ea
	6 ea	5 ea	4 ea
	LATERAL LUNGE—HORIZONTAL RESISTANCE (SLIDE)		
	8 ea	6 ea	5 ea
	8 ea	6 ea	5 ea
	LATERAL PILLAR BRIDGE TO ROW—WITH HIP FLEXION		
	8 ea	10 ea	12 ea
	8 ea	10 ea	12 ea
	REVERSE LUNGE—HORIZONTAL RESISTANCE (SLIDE)		
	8 ea	6 ea	5 ea
	8 ea	6 ea	5 ea
	PILLAR BRIDGE—DYNAMIC ALTERNATING (ARMS IN TRX)		
	8 ea	10 ea	12 ea
	8 ea	10 ea	12 ea

ESD	**150-YARD SHUTTLE**					
	2x6	60 sec rest	2x7	45 sec rest	2x8	30 sec Rest

RG — Soft Tissue Routine
Cold Tub/Compression Boots

POWER B

	Movement	Sets	Reps
PP	Standing Toe Taps	2	5 ea
	Step to Inverted Hamstring Stretch	2	6 ea
	Sidelying Quad/Hip Flexor Stretch w/Rotation	2	4x3 breaths ea
	Supine fallout at 90 Hip flexion with FL connect	2	6 ea
	Fencing Stretch	2	6 ea
MP	Leg Cradle	1	5 ea
	Dropstep Squat	1	5 ea
	Drop Lunge	1	5 ea
	Handwalk	1	5
	Pillar March—Lateral	2	10 steps ea
	Pillar Skip—Lateral	3	10 steps ea
MB	Chest Pass—Standing	3	10 ea
	Overhead Throw	3	10 ea
	Perpendicular Rotational Throw—Standing	3	10 ea

RP	Week 1	Week 2	Week 3
	BOX JUMP (WEIGHT VEST)		
	Quadruped Rocking		
	4	5	6
	4	5	6
	4	5	6

	Week 1	Week 2	Week 3
	PULL UP (10x)		
	*Overhead Slam (MB)		x4
	Reach, Roll, and Lift— Heel Sit (Foam Roll)		x6
	6	5	4
	5*	4*	3*
	5*	4*	3*
	5*	4*	3*
	BENCH PRESS (BARBELL OR DUMBELL) (10x)		
	*Push-Up on Bench-Countermovement (Plyo)		x4
	Sliding Overhead Press		x6
	6	5	4
	5*	4*	3*
	5*	4*	3*
	5*	4*	3*

	Week 1	Week 2	Week 3
	ROTATIONAL CHOP-1 ARM, STANDING, REACTIVE (xxx)		
	Supine Hip Rotator Stretch		x6
	6 ea	5 ea	4 ea
	6 ea	5 ea	4 ea
	ROTATIONAL ROW (TRX)		
	8 ea	6 ea	5 ea
	8 ea	6 ea	5 ea
	PRONE KNEE TUCK (TRX)		
	8	10	12
	8	10	12
	PUSH-UP (TRX)		
	8	6	5
	8	6	5
	90-90 STRETCH WITH ARM SWEEP		
	6ea	6ea	6ea
	6ea	6ea	6ea

ESD	**LADDER SHUTTLE DRILL (5-10-15)**					
	2x6	60 sec rest	2x8	45 sec rest	2x10	30 sec rest

RG — Soft Tissue Routine
Cold Tub/Compression Boots

POWER C

	Movement	Sets	Reps
PP	Inverted Hamstring	1	5 ea
	Leg Cradle	1	5 ea
	Knee Hug	1	5 ea
	Lateral Lunge	1	5 ea
	Reverse Lunge—Forearm to Instep with Rotation	1	5 ea
	Dropstep Skip	3	10 steps ea
PL	Lateral Hurdle Hop—Continuous (Weight Vest)	2	6 ea
	Squat Jump—CM (Weight Vest)	2	4
MB	Walking Lunge to Chest Pass	2	5 ea
	Parallel Rotational Throw—Standing	3	10 ea
	Perpendicular Rotational Throw—Standing	2	10 ea
	Granny Toss	3	5

RP	Week 1	Week 2	Week 3

	Week 1	Week 2	Week 3
	BENT-OVER ROW—1 ARM, 1 LEG (DB—CONTRALATERAL) (10x)		
	Foam Roll—Latissimus Dorsi		x20 sec ea
	6 ea	5 ea	4 ea
	6 ea	5 ea	4 ea
	6 ea	5 ea	4 ea
	SPLIT SQUAT—BACK FOOT ELEVATED (10x)		
	Foam Roll—Quadriceps		x20 sec ea
	6 ea	5 ea	4 ea
	6 ea	5 ea	4 ea
	6 ea	5 ea	4 ea
	BENCH PRESS—1 ARM (DB) (10x)		
	Foam Roll—Chest		x20 sec ea
	6 ea	5 ea	4 ea
	6 ea	5 ea	4 ea
	6 ea	5 ea	4 ea
	RDL—1 ARM, 1 LEG (DB—CONTRALATERAL) (10x)		
	Foam Roll—Hamstring		x20 sec ea
	6 ea	5 ea	4 ea
	6 ea	5 ea	4 ea
	6 ea	5 ea	4 ea

	Week 1	Week 2	Week 3
	ROTATIONAL PUSH/PULL—REACTIVE (xxx)		
	90-90 Stretch with Arm Sweep		x6
	6 ea	5 ea	4 ea
	6 ea	5 ea	4 ea
	PULL-UP		
	6	8	10
	6	8	10
	LATERAL LUNGE—ALTERNATING (DB)		
	6 ea	8 ea	10 ea
	6 ea	8 ea	10 ea
	INCLINE BENCH PRESS—ALTERNATING (DB)		
	6 ea	8 ea	10 ea
	6 ea	8 ea	10 ea
	LEG CURL—1 LEG (SLIDE)		
	6 ea	8 ea	10 ea
	6 ea	8 ea	10 ea

ESD	**50-YARD SPRINTS**					
	2x8	30 sec rest	2x10	30 sec rest	2x12	30 sec rest

RG — Soft Tissue Routine
Cold Tub/Compression Boots

Movement Skills Sessions

MOVEMENT SKILLS—LINEAR

	Movement	Sets	Reps
PP	Foam Roll—Glutes	1	30 sec ea
	Foam Roll—IT Band	1	30 sec ea
	Foam Roll—Quadriceps	1	30 sec ea
	Foam Roll—Latissimus Dorsi	1	30 sec ea
	Trigger Point—Arch/Plantar Fascia	1	50 ea
MP	Miniband Walking—Linear Bent Knee	1	5 ea
	Knee Hug	1	5 ea
	Reverse Lunge—Forearm to Instep with Rotation	1	5 ea
	Drop Lunge	1	5 ea
	Pillar March—Linear	2	10 steps ea
	Pillar Skip—Linear	3	10 steps ea
	2-Inch Runs—In Place	3	6 sec
PL	Horizontal Jump	3	5
	Linear Bound—Quick and Stabilize	2	5 ea
MS	Acceleration Wall Drill—Posture Hold	2	30 sec ea
	Acceleration Wall Drill—Load and Lift	2	8 ea
	Acceleration Wall Drill—Single Exchange	2	8 ea
	Acceleration Sled Drill—Sprint	3	15 yd
	Accelerations	2	15 yd
	Acceleration Sled Drill—Sprint	3	15 yd
	Accelerations	4	15 yd
	Sprint	2	40 yd
	Sled March—Low	4	25 yd
ESD	Your Choice	2 to 3	5 min Hard/1 min Easy
RG	Soft Tissue Routine		
	Cold Tub or Compression Boots	1	20min

MOVEMENT SKILLS—COMBINATION

	Movement	Sets	Reps
PP	Foam Roll—Glutes	1	30 sec ea
	Foam Roll—IT Band	1	30 sec ea
	Foam Roll—Quadriceps	1	30 sec ea
	Foam Roll—Latissimus Dorsi	1	30 sec ea
	Trigger Point—Arch/Plantar Fascia	1	50 ea
MP	Miniband Walking—Linear, Bent Knee	1	5 ea
	Knee Hug	1	5 ea
	Reverse Lunge—Forearm to Instep with Rotation	1	5 ea
	Drop Lunge	1	5 ea
	Lateral Lunge	1	5 ea
	Pillar March—Linear	2	10 steps ea
	Pillar Skip—Lateral	3	10 steps ea
	2-Inch Runs—In Place	3	6 sec
PL	Horizontal Jump	3	5
	Rotational Bound—90 deg Quick and Stabilize	3	5 ea
MS	Acceleration Wall Drill—Single Exchange	2	8 ea
	Acceleration Sled Drill—Sprint	3	15 yd
	Accelerations	2	15 yd
	Lateral Shuffle—Resisted Continuous	3	3 ea
	Lateral Shuffle—Continuous	3	3 ea
	Sprints	2	40 yd
	Sled March—Low	4	25 yd
ESD	Your Choice	2 to 3	5 min Hard/1 min Easy
RG	Soft Tissue Routine		
	Cold Tub or Compression Boots	1	20 min

MOVEMENT SKILLS—MULTIDIRECTIONAL

	Movement	Sets	Reps
PP	5-Way Hip Cable	1	10 ea
MP	Miniband Walking—Lateral, Bent Knee	1	10 steps ea
	Lateral Lunge	1	5 ea
	Leg Cradle	1	5 ea
	Handwalk	1	5
	Crossover Skip	2	10 steps ea
	Tinioca	2	10 steps ea
	Dropstep Skip	3	10 steps ea
	Base Rotations	3	6 sec
PL	Rotational Bound—90 deg Quick and Stabilize	3	5 ea
MS	Crossover Drill—Quick and Stabilze	2	6 ea
	Crossover Drill—Resisted Continuous	4	3 ea
	Lateral Shuffle—Resisted Quick and Stabilize	3	3 ea
	Lateral Shuffle—Quick and Stabilize	1	3 ea
	Lateral Shuffle—Resisted Continuous	3	3 ea
	Lateral Shuffle—Continuous	3	3 ea
ESD	Your Choice	2 to 3	30 sec Sprint/4:30 min Hard/ 2min Easy
RG	Soft Tissue Routine		
	Cold Tub or Compression Boots	1	20min

Regeneration Sessions

GENERAL REGENERATION

	Movement	Sets	Reps
ESD	Your Choice	1	20 min Easy
RG	Trigger Point—Thoracic Spine	1	5 ea
	Trigger Point—Glutes	4	45 sec ea
	Trigger Point—TFL	1	45 sec ea
	Trigger Point—Neck	1	45 sec
	Foam Roll—Upper Back	1	45 sec
	Foam Roll—Low Back	1	45 sec ea
	Foam Roll—Glutes	1	45 sec ea
	Foam Roll—IT Band	1	45 sec ea
	Foam Roll—Quadriceps	1	45 sec ea
	Reach, Roll, and Lift—Heel Sit (Foam Roll)	1	10
	Bent Knee Hamstring Stretch	1	10 ea
	Abductor Stretch—Rope	1	10 ea

FLEXIBILITY

	Movement	Sets	Reps
ESD	Your Choice	1	20 min Easy
RG	Trigger Point—Arch/Plantar Fascia	2	50 ea
	Reach, Roll, and Lift—Heel Sit (Foam Roll)	2	10
	Bent Knee Hamstring Stretch	2	10 ea
	Abductor Stretch—Supine (Rope)	2	10 ea
	Supine Hip Internal Rotation Stretch	2	10 ea
	Quad Hip Flexor Stretch—1/2 Kneeling	2	10 ea
	90—90 Stretch with Arm Sweep	2	10 ea
	Sidelying Shoulder Stretch	2	10 ea
	Quad/Hip Flexor Stretch—Sidelying	2	10 ea

LOW BACK PAIN

	Movement	Sets	Reps
ESD	Your Choice	1	20 min Easy
RG	Trigger Point—Thoracic Spine	1	5 ea
	Massage Stick—Low Back	1	45 sec
	Trigger Point—Glutes	1	45 sec ea
	Trigger Point—TFL	1	45 sec ea
	Foam Roll—Thoracic Spine	2	45 sec
	Foam Roll—Low Back	2	45 sec ea
	Foam Roll—Glutes	2	45 sec ea
	Foam Roll—Hamstrings	2	45 sec ea
	Foam Roll—Quadriceps	2	45 sec ea
	Reach, Roll, and Lift—Heel Sit (Foam Roll)	2	10
	Bent Knee Hamstring Stretch	2	10 ea
	Quad/Hip Flexor Stretch—Half Kneeling	2	10 ea
	90-90 Stretch with Arm Sweep	2	10 ea

KNEE PAIN

	Movement	Sets	Reps
ESD	Your Choice	1	20 min Easy
RG	Massage Stick—Quadriceps	1	45 sec ea
	Massage Stick—Hamstrings	1	45 sec ea
	Massage Stick—TFL	1	45 sec ea
	Trigger Point—Glutes	1	45 sec ea
	Trigger Point—VMO	1	10 ea
	Trigger Point—TFL	1	45 sec ea
	Foam Roll—Glutes	2	45 sec ea
	Foam Roll—Hamstrings	2	45 sec ea
	Foam Roll—IT Band	2	45 sec ea
	Foam Roll—Quadriceps	2	45 sec ea
	Foam Roll—Adductor	2	45 sec ea
	Foam Roll—Tibialis Anterior	2	45 sec

SELF MASSAGE

	Movement	Sets	Reps
ESD	Your Choice	1	20 min Easy
RG	Trigger Point—Thoracic Spine	1	5 ea
	Trigger Point—Glutes	4	45 sec ea
	Trigger Point—TFL	1	45 sec ea
	Trigger Point—VMO	2	10 ea
	Trigger Point—Arch/Plantar Fascia	1	50 ea
	Trigger Point—Neck	1	45 sec
	Foam Roll—Thoracic Spine	1	45 sec
	Foam Roll—Low Back	1	45 sec ea
	Foam Roll—Glutes	1	45 sec ea
	Foam Roll—Hamstrings	1	45 sec ea
	Foam Roll—Calf	1	45 sec ea
	Foam Roll—Quadriceps	1	45 sec ea
	Foam Roll—Adductor	1	45 sec ea

UPPER BACK/SHOULDER PAIN

	Movement	Sets	Reps
ESD	Your Choice	1	20 min Easy
RG	Massage Stick—Neck	1	45 sec
	Trigger Point—Thoracic Spine	1	5 ea
	Trigger Point—Neck	1	45 sec
	Foam Roll—Thoracic Spine	2	45 sec
	Foam Roll—Low Back	2	45 sec ea
	Foam Roll—Latissimus Dorsi	2	45 sec ea
	Foam Roll—Chest	2	45 sec ea
	Reach, Roll, and Lift—Heel Sit (Foam Roll)	2	10
	Sidelying Shoulder Stretch	2	10 ea

HIP PAIN

	Movement	Sets	Reps
ESD	Your Choice	1	20 min Easy
RG	Massage Stick—TFL	1	45 sec ea
	Trigger Point—Glutes	1	45 sec ea
	Foam Roll—Glutes	2	45 sec ea
	Foam Roll—Hamstrings	2	45 sec ea
	Foam Roll—IT Band	2	45 sec ea
	Foam Roll—Quadriceps	2	45 sec ea
	Bent Knee Hamstring Stretch	2	10 ea
	Abductor Stretch—Rope	2	10 ea
	Supine Hip Internal Rotation Stretch	2	10 ea
	Quad/Hip Flexor Stretch—Half Kneeling	2	10 ea

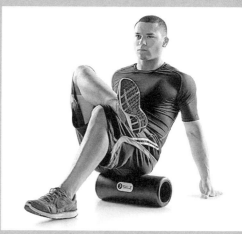

4 | REST FOR IT

Athletes' Performance Recovery

ONE OF THE CORNERSTONES OF THE ATHLETES' PERFORMANCE PROGRAM, THE element that perhaps separates us from fitness programs, diets, and other training regimens, is our emphasis on recovery.

If we wanted to make you throw up in six seconds with a training session, we could do that. That's not our goal, however. We want to create a sustainable system of high performance. And we do that by being precise in every aspect of recovery between sets, reps, sessions, days, and weeks through working recovery into every aspect of your lifestyle, from the minute you wake up to when you go to bed. If you don't, you stand no chance in elevating your performance for the long haul.

This is not just about taking a day off from training once or twice a week or getting an occasional massage, both of which are effective strategies. Instead, when we talk about recovery, we're referring to a number of methods you use over the course of the day to fuel your success.

After all, it's impossible to go all out all the time. Your mind and body require time to recover. Recovery is the limiting factor to performance and in performance training. If you could recover immediately at the highest quality, you could get right back out there and train harder, longer, and faster.

This is impossible, of course. You can't continue to go harder and harder without giving your mind and body time to adapt from the training stimulus. Look at this recovery time as the equivalent of recharging your batteries or refueling your tank. If you recognize and follow this simple formula, you will dramatically increase performance. The ability to take advantage of this window, shrinking the time to achieve full recovery, dictates how close you are to being the best at what you do.

WORK + REST = SUCCESS

Work is the stress that is placed on the mind and body. Recovery is the limiting factor of any training system. No matter how well you follow the training portion of the program, your success will be compromised if you don't have adequate recovery.

If you followed our Core Performance books, this concept might sound familiar. But like everything else in this program, we've stepped it up a notch. Recovery is not just what you do postworkout or on recovery days. It's a 24/7 process. As you'll learn in this section, it involves going through a sleep ritual to ensure that you get the most out of your slumber. It includes soft tissue and trigger point movements throughout the course of the day, not just at designated portions of the training sessions. Recovery involves a daily power nap, breathing techniques, and hydrotherapy. And as discussed in the Nutrition section, we also fuel for recovery all day.

Recovery is such an important, integrated part of this program that you will eat, breathe, and sleep recovery.

That's because the things you do to promote recovery are just as important as the work you perform. If you focus on having high-quality recovery, you'll be able to get more return on your investment from every waking moment of duty or training.

These recovery strategies will increase energy, boost your immune system, and help you get the most out of each day and each training session, which ultimately will improve your performance. Recovery will improve your hormone profile, decrease inflammation, and improve tissue quality, thus decreasing the number of overuse injuries you may experience.

Recovery strategies apply to every aspect of your life. In the United States, we've developed such a workaholic mentality that we've become inefficient. We work so hard, with so little time to recover, that our productivity suffers, and ultimately we break down. We want to be more efficient and enjoy all aspects of our lives. Recovery helps that happen.

In previous books we used the words *recovery* and *regeneration* interchangeably. The idea was that *recovery* refers to the actual process of physically and psychologically overcoming the stresses of preparation, while *regeneration* refers to the activities or strategies to help jump-start recovery.

Here we've integrated this into a complete mindset of Recovery. That's why we talk about recovering *for* it rather than *from* it. When we look at recovery as simply a post-training strategy, we limit our mindset to how we rebound from training, action, or heavy activity. It becomes more of a one-dimensional postworkout and day-after philosophy.

But when we think in terms of "Rest for It," we're now acting at a higher level. The idea is that these strategies employed over the course of the day aren't just helping us recover physically and mentally, but they're keeping us operating at the highest possible level to help us fuel that IT, the grand vision for our lives.

It all starts with the confidence to know that reloading your gun is not a waste of time, but a necessity if you want to continue to fire rounds of excellence. Focusing on the body, we need to understand that how we treat our soft tissue, our fascia, is critical to our approach. The quality of your muscles and fascia is directly related to the quality of your overall approach to recovery and training.

When we talk about the tissue, we're referring not just to muscle but all the fascia and connective tissue throughout your body. The fascia are intricate systems that organize your body and all your muscles into multiplanar slings that optimize movement.

We need to look at the fascia and the muscle as interrelated systems. Some of the recovery techniques we will use will be targeted toward the changing of fascial length and pliability, and others at the mind and muscle. Think of fascia as a plastic-type substance that will take more time to adapt to the stimulus.

Examples of how we'll change fascia include elements of static stretching (when your body is cold and not warmed up) and elements of self-massage, as well as work with massage therapists. We'll work on this throughout the day, from when we wake up to when we go to bed over the course of our Performance Day.

The second layer of your tissue quality will be addressing the muscle living within this fascial system. Through training inefficient movement patterns and the demands of your sport and equipment, your muscles likely have become shortened and stiff. You will learn how to move efficiently, which paired with proper recovery will allow your muscles to lengthen and become more pliable and elastic.

Let's take a look at these Recovery strategies.

ATHLETES' PERFORMANCE RECOVERY

1. Fuel
2. Sleep
3. Breathe
4. Hydrotherapy
5. Self-Massage
6. Stretching

1 | Fuel

We discussed this at length in the Nutrition section, but it bears repeating that we're not just fueling for performance, we're also fueling to recover. By consuming nutrient-dense, fiber-rich, high-performance power foods every three hours, we're ensuring that we're able to thrive all day despite all the stresses that are thrown at us.

2 | Sleep

Sleep is a vital component of recovery. It rebuilds the brain and body, releasing rejuvenating hormones, and allows us to stay focused throughout the day, hitting the brain's "refresh" button.

In 2001, the National Sleep Foundation performed its famous "Sleep in America" survey, determining that 63 percent of adults get less than the recommended eight hours of sleep per night and 31 percent get less than seven hours. More than 40 percent of adult Americans reported having trouble staying awake during the day.

Sleep deprivation can interfere with memory, energy levels, cognition, and mood. Without sleep you cannot function at your best. Sleep debt undermines your ability to eat healthfully and train as well, thus raising your level of body fat. When the brain is exhausted, it doesn't know whether it's sleep-deprived or starving for glucose, so the natural response is to crave sugar, which is why you have late-night cravings when you're tired. When you're low on energy, your body wants to conserve it, so motivation to train is greatly reduced.

Sleep is the magic pill. No one would argue that sleep upgrades nearly all systems and is the foundation of high performance.

During sleep your brain has the ability to repair, restore, and lock in all that you've learned that day. Your body does the same. This is where the majority of your hormones, such as growth hormone and testosterone, are released. It's when your fascia, muscles, and neuromuscular system go through an upgrading from the stimulus you gave it earlier.

Sleep is like everything else in your life; it's a skill. Getting a great night's sleep is a skill you can and must develop. Our athletes get so passionate about this. They know it's one area where they can drastically improve performance without necessarily putting forth greater physical effort or resources.

So what makes a successful night's sleep? How do you know if your brain and body had an overnight upgrade and will be ready to achieve today at a higher level? How can you make sure you wake up with the energy, vitality, and positive outlook necessary to achieve today?

First, it's necessary to learn about sleep cycles. Sleep is broken down into cycles consisting of varying depths of sleep. The three main categories are light sleep, REM sleep, and deep sleep.

The initial stage of sleep is light sleep, followed after about ninety minutes by REM (rapid eye movement). REM sleep is critical for brain performance and for organizing memory to better apply what you learn. REM sleep is where the brain upgrades from the stimulus of the day. When you're able to get high-quality REM sleep, you wake up refreshed and refocused.

Whereas REM sleep helps above the neck, deep sleep helps below the neck, upgrading your body. This is an oversimplification, as obviously this is an integrated system. Deep sleep releases the growth hormone and testosterone necessary for your body to recover from the stimulation you gave it during the day. This results in support of your lean body mass, decreases in your body fat, and an overall improved recovery of all your body's physical systems. Deep sleep is important for restoring muscle and building immunity.

You cannot perform at the highest level without great sleep. Sleep cycles range from between 90 to 120 minutes. Your body cycles from light to REM to deep sleep and back to light sleep. You go through between three and five cycles of sleep per night, depending on the amount of time asleep.

The foundation to great sleep is consistency, getting between seven and nine hours of sleep a night during the same time frame. High achievers sometimes pride themselves on how they're able to operate on little sleep. That's a mistake. You must be a better manager of your time and performance, and this starts with sleep. If you choose to prioritize other things over sleep, you are deficit-spending with your performance and health.

In an ideal world, you'd go to sleep at the same time each night, so that your body can continue to build a rhythm to your day and ultimately to your sleep. The more sleep you get *before* midnight, the better night sleep you will receive. You'll undergo more REM and deep sleep, releasing more positive hormones.

Don't assume that sleeping from midnight to nine a.m. is equivalent to sleeping from nine p.m. to six a.m. They leave you in two different states of rest (or unrest).

Length of sleep is always debated. It's more important to be consistent. If that means seven hours, be consistent with seven hours. That's because the body likes consistency. The body needs to know it can count on you to be consistent in letting it know how much time it has to undergo this overnight upgrade. Just as you always want to know how long work or an athletic practice is going to last, your body wants to know how long it has for sleep. Once you've installed that consistent window for sleep, the body is able to establish its own game plan for how long it will stay in each sleep cycle and make sure you wake up at the top of your sleep cycle each morning.

The body is amazing at adapting based on the situation that you give it. If you got seven hours of sleep, seven nights per week, your body will be in a far better state than if you were to get ten hours one night, four the next, six the following, and eleven the night after that. We know our elite clients have random and chaotic schedules dictated by their employers, but to have this consistent sleep length and ritual will anchor your success. You might have some thirty-six-hour days, and you'll perform, but when we shut down, work this ritual, your mind and body know they need to immediately go to work during this window.

Eight hours is considered the gold standard for sleep. The National Institutes of Health (NIH) recommend seven to nine hours of sleep for adults regardless of age, though people typically get less than that.

Length of sleep changes as you age. In your twenties, you'll average 7.3 hours, with about 1.6 hours of REM, 83 minutes of deep sleep, and 16 minutes of time needed to fall asleep. In your thirties, you might average 7.1 hours: 1.5 hours of REM, 69 minutes of deep, and 21 minutes to fall asleep. In your forties, you'll average 6.8 hours: 1.4 hours of REM, 56 minutes of deep, and 28 minutes to fall asleep.

See a pattern? In your fifties, you'll average 6.5 hours of sleep: 1.3 hours of REM, 44 minutes of deep, and 38 minutes to fall asleep. In your sixties, you'll average 6.3 hours of sleep: 1.2 hours of REM, 36 minutes of deep, and 52 minutes to fall asleep. By your seventies, you'll average 6 hours sleep: 1.1 hours of REM, 30 minutes of deep, and 68 minutes to fall asleep.

Ideally you'll sleep through the night in a deep slumber, but there are some people who sleep deeply for four hours, wake for two or three, return to bed for an additional three hours, and still wake feeling very refreshed. I'm not saying this is normal, but these quiet hours after the initial sleep wave are some of the most powerful and insightful hours you might have.

Ideally, elite performers wake up without an alarm clock. The alarm clock is simply there as a backup to your innate circadian rhythm clock. When you rely on an alarm clock to wake up, it's highly probable that you're being woken up in the middle of a sleep cycle.

If you've ever been woken up in the middle of a deep sleep cycle, you know that disoriented feeling. You don't know where you are and have a hard time recovering from this sluggish feeling for the rest of the day. This is called sleep inertia. You're groggy, not focused, and it just seems to be one of those days. Hitting the snooze button is another way to induce sleep inertia, so when the alarm goes off, get going!

Few people give any thought to a sleep ritual and the impact it has not only on sleep but also on their performance throughout the day.

First create the proper sleep environment. Block all light from the bedroom. This includes artificial nighttime light, everything from external (streetlights, passing car lights) to internal lights (night-lights, clocks). Depending on the time of year, sunlight can wake you prematurely in the early morning hours. So make your bedroom as comfortable as possible by blocking out light sources with blackout curtains or an eye mask.

The Power Nap

Your Performance Day should include a small window for a power nap. Elite performers are great at finding a way to fit this into their schedules. Some of history's most significant figures have taken daily naps, a group that includes Albert Einstein, Napoleon Bonaparte, Sir Isaac Newton, John F. Kennedy, Winston Churchill, and Leonardo da Vinci.

Naps reduce stress, enhance memory, improve stamina, boost creativity, preserve youth, and increase your sex drive. Naps are helpful in weight maintenance and improve your perception and accuracy. And, of course, naps feel good.

As kindergartners we learn the restorative powers of a nap, placing our heads on our desks or lying on a mat. Unfortunately we quickly break this powerful habit. An afternoon siesta of just twenty to thirty minutes can give you a second wind for the rest of the day. It's part of European culture not just because of tradition, but because it's so effective.

Find a way to get horizontal (on your back) with your feet up for twenty to thirty minutes. Power naps are a skill. The first time you start to power nap, you will have a difficult time disassociating from the demand of your day to getting to a restful state. Don't worry; you too can master this skill. Relax, be patient with yourself and, if nothing else, spending twenty to thirty minutes with your eyes closed, with your body relaxed, and trying to quiet your mind through breathing techniques—breathing in for a count of four, holding for two, and exhaling for a six count (4-2-6 breathing)—will result in a higher level performance later. Think of this as an opportunity to do a quick recharge on your brain and on your body, allowing you to leave the power nap with greater focus and greater energy to continue to achieve.

The goal of the power nap is to go from light to REM sleep and pull out of it in just twenty to thirty minutes, leaving your body thinking it just went through a full sleep cycle. This is what helps restore the brain and will improve your focus, your ability to learn and apply. These twenty- to thirty-minute naps can add up to three and a half hours of sleep a week.

Perhaps you're worried that you won't wake up from your power nap for hours. If that happens, you're probably not getting enough sleep. Set an alarm on your mobile device for backup if you'd like. Or take some caffeine immediately before your nap, perhaps as part of your midafternoon fueling.

Taking caffeine might seem counterintuitive to napping. But the caffeine won't hit you for twenty to thirty minutes, so you'll wake up from REM sleep and get an additional boost from the caffeine, allowing you to perform at an even higher level. Caffeine also causes micromuscle contractions, which help keep the muscles toned while you nap.

Power naps are a skill that will take some time to develop. If getting horizontal isn't realistic, consider getting a quick nap on the plane, bus, or train (taking safety into account). Take advantage of wherever you can get a quick reload.

During one research study, college students were not allowed to sleep but were given a chance to power nap every four hours. The kids made it more than twenty days before they collapsed. Such experimentation could occur only with college students, of course, but it does show the power of naps to reset the brain and continue to sustain the body without the great deep sleep we discussed above. It also shows that you'll fail without deep sleep, let alone thrive to the level we expect. Special Forces operatives who seldom get the right amount of restful sleep use naps to keep at their peaks, and it works that way for everyone.

Breathe in calming scents. Smelling aromatherapy oils or lotions in calming scents like chamomile or lavender helps relax the brain and leads to deeper sleep. Try a heat diffuser or place calming scents on or near your pillow.

Chill out at night. Lower your thermostat before you go to bed. Cooler temperatures have been shown to help you sleep longer and more soundly.

Next, follow a sleep ritual:

—Power down to relax. Electronics keep your brain busy. Remove all electronic devices (phone, television, laptops, tablets) from your bedroom and see how your sleep improves.

—Thirty minutes before bedtime, practice a few calming activities: drink a cup of herbal tea, stretch, meditate, or read a short inspirational story (no reading the news before bedtime). After a few weeks, this will become habit, and you'll fall asleep faster.

—Focus on the positive. Negativity can drag you down and put a damper on your day. If you struggle with negative thoughts, think of three positive things that happened to you that day. As you focus on the positive events of your day, your thoughts will begin to shift. Review the positives of your Performance Day. Visualize the benefits of living your IT and all for which you are grateful.

—Create a quiet place. Listen to some relaxing music to drown out outside noise or use a white noise machine. Practice clearing your thoughts and focus on your breathing once you go to bed. Give thanks as you do your calming 6-4-10 breathing practice. Inhale through your nose for six counts, hold for four counts, and then exhale through your nose for ten counts. Repeat ten times to relax your mind and body and induce sleep.

3 | Breathe

Now that we've convinced you that you've been sleeping ineffectively all your life, we'll show you how you haven't been breathing effectively, either.

The average person takes more than eight million breaths a year, and yet chances are you have not been breathing for high performance.

If there were a movement pattern you did twenty-three thousand times a day, you no doubt would take measures to improve it. But how often do you consider your breathing? The majority of athletes we see have such dysfunctional breathing patterns that it limits their performance, increases potential for injury, and often has them all worked up psychologically.

Perhaps you think you understand proper breathing from squatting or bench pressing in the gym. You know to breathe in as a weight is lowered, pause, and then exhale as the weight is raised.

That's the process, to be sure, but it's just a small part of your day. We're talking breathing from the moment you wake up to the moment you go to bed as well as when you sleep. This all-day breathing affects your body's ability to recover, your anatomical structure, your autonomic nervous system (ANS), and your cognitive ability. There are not many skills that can upgrade nearly every aspect of performance.

Many people use only a small percentage of the body's ability to draw oxygenated air into their lungs because they tend to breathe only with the upper part of their torso (chest breathing), instead of deep breathing, which starts at the pelvic floor and works up through the base of the rib cage. Breathing should occur from the action of the diaphragm, the most efficient breathing muscle, and not the accessory muscles of the chest and neck. In general, the rib cage should expand in a 3-D pattern, top to bottom, back to front, and to the sides, acting as a basket that cradles your lungs, not a restricting cage.

To better understand this, lie on your back. Place your right hand with your thumb below your ribs and the center of your palm on your abs as if you had a tummy ache. Put your other hand up on your chest, centered on your ribs.

Inhaling through your nose, pull the breath deep down into your lower abdomen, creating tension under your lower hand and deepening your breath so that you feel the expansion all the way toward your lower back and lower abdominal cavity. This action of the diaphragm lowering toward your pelvis is mirrored by the action of the pelvic floor muscles, enhancing pillar strength while allowing the lungs to completely fill with fresh air. At this point, there should have been minimal movement in your upper hand or chest. Finish the inhalation, then exhale and repeat.

This is a movement skill, no different from any other you've learned in sport or training. Practice it with focus and confidence that you will achieve this. Once you master the skill, it will be one of the more dramatic performance enhancers you can make on and off the field, in and out of competition.

By changing the way you breathe, you will improve your posture and the muscular tone and tissue quality of some of the areas where you likely carry a lot of tension, such as your shoulders, upper back, chest, and neck.

One reason we preach pillar strength and posture frequently is that this foundation allows us to be successful not only at high-performance movements but also with our breathing.

Many athletes have an anterior tilt of their pelvis oriented forward, along with extension of their thoracic spine, making it look like they have a big arch in the back. If you were to draw a line on their lower ribs and the top of their pelvis, it's big and open, like an alligator's mouth ready to strike.

This position with a protruding abdomen does not allow the right type of length/tension relationship for the movement patterns of your sport or mission. The muscles required for breathing need to have the same type of foundation so that they can perform.

High performers take advantage of a deep inhalation and a powerful exhalation. The majority of athletes we see don't have the ability to do either well due to poor posture, which undermines speed, power, endurance, and recovery, as well as cognitive function.

Want to see how well you breathe? Try the following test. Place one hand on your chest and one below your ribs on your stomach. Breathe in deeply. The hand on your chest shouldn't move at all; the hand on your stomach should move out as you breathe in. This means your diaphragm is moving down and outward, sucking air into your chest. Your chest muscles around your ribs and below your neck are strong and tight, so moving them to breathe will zap your energy.

Keeping Your ANS Balanced

The autonomic nervous system (ANS) controls the majority of your body's functions and has two major divisions. The sympathetic nervous system is responsible for stimulating fight-or-flight activities, while the parasympathetic nervous system relates to the "rest and digest" elements that occur while the body is at rest. There is a third division, the enteric system, surrounding your gut with an extensive nervous system that is highly reactive to input from the rest of the body.

In today's fast-paced society, we're always stimulated through technology, stress, caffeine intake, and poor breathing habits. The fight-or-flight response tends to be our default normal state. Now if we look at the added demands placed on those operating in sports and the tactical space, it's easy to see how you could constantly be in an even greater level of sympathetic activity.

That's not where you want to be. This fight-or-flight response was meant for survival purposes, not for steady-state activity. It's not a sustainable situation, let alone an efficient one. The fight-or-flight response stimulates the pituitary gland and releases the stress hormone cortisol, which is highly inflammatory, a true negative for the brain's and body's performance.

To achieve high levels of performance all day, it's important that we balance the autonomic nervous system. We do this by breathing, sleeping, and fueling properly. We manage our energy and mindset throughout the day to apply the highest levels of effort—the fight-or-flight stimulus—only when needed and to return quickly to the parasympathetic "rest and digest" position so that the body is in a state of recovery.

We can use breathing techniques throughout the course of the day to make this happen. Think in terms of a breathing tempo that consists of an inhale, a hold, and an exhale. A tempo of 6-4-10, for instance, means a six-second inhale, a four-second hold, and a ten-second exhale. This will take some training to achieve. Start by utilizing a tempo of 4-2-6 as the faster-paced alternative, which achieves much the same effect. The goal is a longer exhale than inhale. You'll also find this easier if you have been exerting during a game, practice, or training session.

The science behind this is that a long exhale brings the parasympathetic neurons into play. Since cortisol levels peak around four and five a.m., the sympathetic tone is quite high then as well. If you wake up feeling stressed or tired, then use 6-4-10 to relax, or just a quick inhale followed by an explosive exhale to wake you might clear the mind and sharpen you up.

But if you are tired or perhaps hit the

snooze button once or twice, the delta and theta waves of sleep are going to hang around the whole day, producing a groggy feeling you just can't shake. If that's the case, spend a minute or two in a 6-2-X tempo to jump-start your day. The X stands for as fast as possible, an explosive exhale. This explosive exhalation gets rid of any remaining "bad" air and can preload the rib cage for the inhalation so the rib cage is ready to expand for that next breath in. Swimmers and boxers use explosive exhalations to power their movements, as the diaphragm is the biggest muscle in the body.

Breathing can rev you up to peak sharpness as well. You might want to try a 4-0-X to oxygenate your body when you need to get some sharpness going before a session, or if you are feeling fatigued by exercise and need to find more fuel in the tank, helping to get some oxygen to the muscles.

During the day, the 4-2-6 or 6-4-10 breathing tempos calm the nervous system, placing you in a "rest and digest" mode rather than a fight-or-flight response. The "rest and digest" mode also is important before meals. By engaging in breathing tempo, you'll become more mindful of healthful eating by changing the blood flow to your gut, reducing acid, and preparing your body for the upcoming digestion workload.

As you're lying in bed, reflecting and giving thanks for the day, use the 4-2-6 or 6-4-10 tempos to reduce anxiety and better prepare yourself for quality sleep. These tempos also work should you awaken at four a.m., when cortisol is rising. The breathing will help you get back to sleep. You can use these two last tempos in the bus on the way to the game, helping keep you in a calm, restful state prior to the explosive launch of power that the adrenaline starting the game will provide. The table on page 128 summarizes the various tempos you can try out.

Practicing diaphragm breathing is easy. Breathe out all the way. While holding your empty lungs, count out loud, "One, two, three, four," until your voice fades because there is no air. Hold on as long as you can until your body automatically forces your lungs open. You will see your stomach pop out as the phrenic nerve forces the diaphragm to move down and suck air in. Do this a few times and you will feel the difference, powering your breathing and saving you energy.

Performance Breathing Chart

Performance Breathing Chart	
Event	Breathing Tempo • IN-HOLD-EXHALE (Seconds) X = Explosive
Wake Up Tired	6-2-X
Wake Up Anxious	6-4-10
Periodically During Day	4-2-6
Moments of Anxiety	6-4-10
Moments of Tiredness	4-0-X
Meditating	8-4-12
Before Meals	4-2-6
Bedtime	6-4-12

Used with permission—Roy Sugarman, Ph.D.

Much has been written about athletes being "in the zone," this rarefied air where they're clicking on all cylinders. It's the basketball player who hits a dozen shots in a row or a baseball player who is hitting so well that every pitch seems as big as a beach ball. These players are performing subconsciously, flowing in the moment, not even thinking about what they're doing.

Breathing is a big part of being in the zone. If you're engaged in typical shallow breathing through the chest, you're not recovered and you're likely not going to reach that easy flow state regardless of how you're performing. The ability to get that exchange of fresh air into your blood creates that zone. Shallow breathing, meanwhile, drives up blood acidity, that uncomfortable lactate threshold feeling that athletes endure with clouded minds and burning muscles.

Improper breathing increases the time needed for recovery, gets in the way of creating ideal brain performance, and is a sign of an inefficient performer. When we're able to switch toward deep breathing through the lower abdomen, we're allowing for a better respiratory exchange, allowing the athlete to calm down and mentally slow down the game. This will improve your speed, power, and endurance while you maintain greater focus on performing at the highest level with less effort, staying calm under pressure.

In addition, many athletes routinely sabotage performance by listening to high-energy, pounding music before a game to get them pumped. Stadium operators have taken this to an art form, creating playlists that incite both the crowd and the athletes.

We respect the mindset of wanting to get as up as possible and focused in your preperformance rituals. At the same time, when you talk to athletes who have thrived at the highest level, playing in front of crowds of up to a hundred thousand people, they'll often say how they didn't hear the crowd or the music at all. They slowed the game down.

That process begins preperformance, when you're naturally in an amped-up, slightly nervous state. Instead of fueling that state further with intense music and shallow breathing, choose more relaxed music with a slower beat. I'm not suggesting elevator music or easy listening favorites, but rather music that mirrors the deep breathing you'll perform pregame—and increasingly over the course of the day.

I realize this sounds counterintuitive, especially in a culture where rap, techno, club music, and other high-intensity tunes are most popular. But it's next to impossible to engage in the deep abdominal breathing necessary to be a high performer if you don't train yourself to do so, and it's harder to calm your breathing when your music is pumping you up. Once you can accomplish breath control, you'll be able to perform in the most noisy, chaotic environments possible. For our tactical athletes, those who compete on the fields of battle, this concept is second nature. For them, it can be the difference between life and death. For those "only" competing in sport, it's the difference between being an overexcited, less-efficient rookie and a calm, effective veteran performer.

Learning how, when, and at what tempo to breathe can boost your performance. Breathing properly can improve cognition, performance, recovery, and physique. Take breathing breaks throughout the day and in the evening. Use the Performance Breathing Chart for the right strategy at the right time. Combine your breathing and IT visualization ritual together for a brain and body upgrade.

4 | Hydrotherapy

Hydrotherapy, the use of water for recovery, pain relief, and treatment, is used to increase circulation, decrease inflammation, calm the nervous system, decrease stress, and help you rejuvenate. Here are a few guidelines:

Ideally you have access to a "cold plunge" tub of water, 50 to 55 degrees Fahrenheit. Immerse yourself for six minutes for a lean 185- to 200-pound athlete. Our 300-plus pound athletes with higher body fats might stay in for fifteen to twenty minutes to work through their protective body fat, then large muscle mass. This will decrease inflammation and lower core temperature, optimizing the recovery window.

A shower is just as effective. Alternate three minutes of cold plunging/ showering with three to five minutes in a hot tub/shower with the temperature between 100 and 110 degrees Fahrenheit. Alternating between cold and hot stimulates blood flow and muscle recovery with little effort. The cold therapy in particular decreases the natural postworkout muscle inflammation and can be used alone for six to ten minutes immediately after a workout.

When you enter the warm water, the blood flows out to your skin and limbs to increase the surface area through which heat can dissipate—just as your skin flushes when training in the heat. The cold does the opposite, pulling blood away from the skin and limbs and toward the heart, not unlike what happens when your fingers turn blue in extreme cold. After a workout, this contrast stimulates muscle recovery with little effort.

Hot and cold contrasts force your blood to move fast, from deep in your trunk out to your limbs and skin and then back again. That's a good thing on its own, and when you do it immediately after a workout and on Recovery days, you stimulate blood flow and muscle recovery with hardly any effort. (Resistance training and ESD require energy and create tiny microtears in muscle fibers, which your body repairs in between training sessions, leaving your muscles ready to adapt to further training.)

Bathing in mineral salts in water heated to 97 to 104 degrees Fahrenheit increases core temperature and metabolic rate. It also has a flushing and cleansing effect on the body.

5 | Self-Massage

Fascia was once thought to be only the lining of the muscles, but we're actually held together by fascia. Indeed, fascia make up our structure. These sheets and bands of fibrous connective tissue envelop and bind together muscles, organs, and other structures of the body. Fascia stretch and recoil effectively.

Under a microscope, fascia appears like a spiderweb with dew on it. That's because it's made up of free water and bound water, making it hydrophilic, meaning it has a high affinity for water and thrives in a water-filled environment. Take away the water via dehydration and fascia loses the ability to transfer energy and information throughout the system.

Fascia extends into the nucleus of cells and affects DNA. Therefore, you can affect your genetics—positively or negatively—by working on your fascia or choosing to ignore them. Fascia are electrical, living structures throughout the body. They're in the cells of our toes and eyes. They're around our muscles, bones, and organs and also within them.

Fascia house twenty times more proprioceptors than anything else in the body. These small supercomputers, spread throughout the body, react much faster than anything else.

We discussed this in the elasticity portion of the Movement section. Fascia is a great performance enhancer, but we discuss it here because it's also the greatest protector. The reason athletes can land softly after making a leaping catch or enduring a vicious hit is the fascia's ability to react quickly and transfer forces, dissipating energy. Think of how high-tech athletic footwear features suspension elements; fascia provides that naturally.

Everything in this program affects your fascia. It takes six months to make a change in fascial tissue. Under other programs, it could take up to twenty-four months. The reason we can expedite the process is that we're not looking at improving our fascia as something we do only during our one-hour daily workout. If we did, the twenty-four-month timetable would be more realistic. Instead, as with every other aspect of this program, we're going to integrate it over the course of each movement, each day, every day.

Since we have a lot of fascia in our bodies that are responsible for many different things, we're going to break it up and address it in many ways, from movement patterns to hydration, massage, and breathing. Everything we do in this program promotes fascial health and performance.

Two things we'll employ for fascial health and performance are trigger point therapy and self-massage.

TRIGGER POINT EXERCISES

Trigger point exercises work similarly to a foam roller, but they make it easier to isolate and release deeper tissues. You'll use a foot roller, tennis ball, lacrosse ball, or other hard ball for a series of self-massage exercises that work areas such as your IT (iliotibial) band, thoracic spine, and the bottoms of your feet.

One easy way to incorporate trigger point exercises into your Performance Day is to leave a trigger point ball or foot roller by your bathroom vanity. As you brush and floss your teeth each morning and evening, work your feet with the ball or roller, in effect "flossing" your fascia. This is crucial for the health of your feet and lower legs, which are critical to all sport and tactical athletes.

Your hands and feet are the most undertreated parts of your body, and yet they're the most abused. Reflexology researchers believe every body part can be traced to a spot on your hands or feet, so working these areas can have total-body benefits. Treat your hands and feet daily to improve performance, reduce stress, and decrease pain all over.

SELF-MASSAGE

Massage is a powerful way to increase blood flow and circulation to the muscle, improve tissue quality, promote the removal of waste products, increase relaxation, and decrease soreness. There are different types of soft tissue techniques designed to achieve specific effects. These include flushing, trigger point, myofascial, and acupressure.

The length of massage sessions depends on whether the focus is total body or general focus (forty-five to ninety minutes) or an isolated focus (five to thirty minutes), and the sessions can come pre- or post-training, between sessions, or on Regeneration or off days.

If a massage isn't in the budget, use a foam or hard roll to give yourself a massage. Glide your sore muscles over a hard foam roll of tightly packed foam, roughly 5 inches in diameter. We prefer the newer, modern hard rollers that are foam on top of PVC pipe. They tend to last longer and are more effective than traditional foam rollers.

By rotating and rolling your hamstrings, quadriceps, backs, lats, and hips over the foam roll, you will release these spasms and accelerate your body's recovery.

The foam roll routine is like a massage. It uses deep compression to help roll out the muscle spasms that develop during a workout. The compression overstimulates the nerves, signaling the muscle spasm to shut off. This allows the muscles to relax and loosen up, gets the blood and lymphatic system flowing, and helps restore muscles.

You'll probably enjoy the foam roll routine—everyone likes massages. Still, there will be some uncomfortable moments, as there are with a professional massage. Once you're past the first few weeks, though, it will become considerably easier and more comfortable. The foam roll is a great barometer of the quality of your muscle and fascia. The better it feels and the less it hurts, the better the quality of your muscle and fascia.

As you roll on the foam, discovering muscle spasms and pressure points, you'll knead out the knots by working back and forth for thirty to sixty seconds and then holding on that pressure point for an additional thirty seconds until the muscle cries for mercy and releases from spasm.

Another key item in your performance arsenal will be a massage stick, an 18- to 24-inch plastic, beaded stick you'll use for specific self-massage during warm-up, between-set movements, cool-down, and at other times over the course of the day. With the massage stick, you will specifically target your neck, forearms, calves, and lower legs. It will loosen muscles, decrease tension, and reduce headaches.

6 | Stretching

After any training or massage session, the muscle should go through a full range of motion to promote blood flow and waste product removal. Stretching will have two main effects on the muscles and joints: flexibility and mobility.

Flexibility is defined as an improved range of motion *around* a joint, whereas mobility is defined as improved range of motion *within* a joint.

There are three types of stretches that can be used: dynamic, Active Isolated, and static.

DYNAMIC STRETCHING

Dynamic stretching involves the use of basic movement patterns (e.g., the backward lunge) for the purpose of improving flexibility/mobility and preparing the body to train. It also improves stability and coordination. Each stretch can be repeated for 4 to 6 reps. (Note: While this might sound like it belongs more in the Movement section, dynamic stretching can and should be performed on active recovery days.)

ACTIVE ISOLATED STRETCHING

Active Isolated Stretching (AIS) is similar to dynamic stretching and can be used during both Pillar Prep and Regeneration sessions. This type of stretching uses a process called reciprocal inhibition to create length in the muscle the same way we do during movement. Reciprocal inhibition is a fancy way of saying that when one muscle group contracts, the other relaxes. When one fires, the other reloads. More than working your muscles, you're reprogramming your brain.

Active Isolated Stretching, developed by Aaron Mattes to target specific muscles that get short or stiff from the demands of life, will help you dramatically increase your flexibility. The key to AIS is its *active* nature. To perform the stretches, you won't stretch for ten to thirty seconds, as in traditional stretching. Instead, you'll hold each stretch for just one or two seconds, thus increasing the muscles' range of motion a few more degrees with each repetition, reprogramming your muscles to contract and relax through new ranges of motion. Exhale during the hold position, releasing tension and getting a deeper stretch. Return to the starting position and repeat for the desired number of reps. This type of exercise requires you to put your "mind in the muscle" to focus on firing the proper muscles and relaxing the muscles to be stretched.

You can do AIS exercises using an 8- to 10-foot length of rope, about the thickness of a jump rope. Go to a home improvement store and have a length cut off for just a few dollars. Wrap the rope around one foot at a time and perform a series of movements that will improve your flexibility. For example, to stretch your hamstring, lie on your back with a rope wrapped around the arch of your right foot. Lift your leg as far as you can into the air, pull your toe up toward your shin, then squeeze or fire your quadriceps, hip flexors, and abs. Give gentle assistance by pulling on the rope and then holding for two seconds. Return to the starting position and continue for 8 to 10 repetitions.

STATIC STRETCHING

Static stretching is a great tool to use during Recovery sessions. This type of stretching is effective for decreasing muscle spasms. The stretches used in Active Isolated Stretching also can be used in static stretching, but without any activation. These stretches are therefore passive and are great for recovery.

Each static stretch can be held for forty-five to sixty seconds, allowing for the muscles to relax. As a rule of thumb, avoid static stretching prior to working out—static stretching works by putting the muscle and the nervous system in a submissive hold until it shuts off and releases. Static stretching should be limited to postworkout and days off.

On Regeneration days, you might want to do extended static stretching sessions consisting of holds of up to three minutes each combined with your deep-breathing activities. Normally this will happen after some warm-up, which will increase your range of motion. Yoga is a complementary activity to achieve many of these benefits. Build static stretching into your day, first or last thing, and throughout your week.

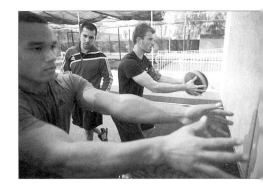

Athletes' Performance Movement Library

5-Way Hip Cable

STEPS

ADDUCTION

1. Attach an ankle strap to the low pulley of a cable machine and stand perpendicular to the machine with the strap attached to your inside ankle.
2. Keeping your leg straight, slowly sweep your inside leg toward your outside leg.
3. Maintaining your balance, return to the starting position and continue for the prescribed number of repetitions.

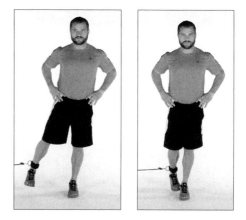

FLEXION

4. Rotate 90 degrees so that you are standing on one leg facing away from the machine in a quarter squat.
5. Lift the knee of the leg with the ankle strap up in front of your body as you stand tall.
6. Maintaining your balance, return to the starting position and continue for the prescribed number of repetitions.

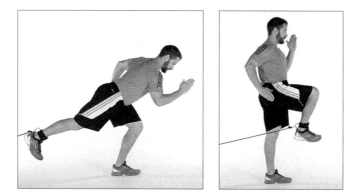

ABDUCTION

7. Rotate another 90 degrees so that you are perpendicular to the machine with the strap on your outside ankle.

8. Keeping your leg straight, slowly move your outside leg out to the side away from your body.

9. Maintaining your balance, return to the starting position and continue for the prescribed number of repetitions.

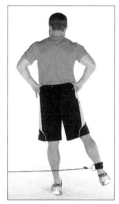

COACHING KEY
Stand tall with your chest up. Stay balanced with good posture without allowing motion to occur at your spine.

FEEL IT
Working your hips and challenging your balance.

EXTENSION

10. Rotate another 90 degrees so that you are standing on one leg facing the machine.

11. Keeping your leg straight, slowly move it backward.

12. Maintaining your balance, return to the starting position and continue for the prescribed number of repetitions.

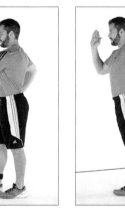

CROSSOVER

13. Rotate another 90 degrees so that you are perpendicular to the machine with the strap on your inside ankle.

14. Balancing on your outside leg, lift your inside knee up and across the front of your body.

15. Maintaining your balance, return to the starting position and continue for the prescribed number of repetitions.

16. Switch legs and repeat the series on your opposite leg.

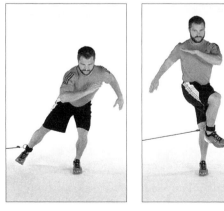

Deep Squat to Hamstring Stretch

COACHING KEY

Keep your arms straight, back flat, and chest up throughout the movement.

FEEL IT

Stretching your glutes and hamstrings.

STEPS

1. Stand tall with your feet wider than hip-width apart.
2. Bend forward at your waist to grab your toes with your hands.
3. Drop down into a deep squat while keeping your arms straight, elbows inside your knees, back flat, and chest up.
4. While holding your toes, raise your hips back and straighten your knees until you feel a good stretch in the back of your legs. Hold for 1 to 2 seconds.
5. Continue for the remainder of the set.

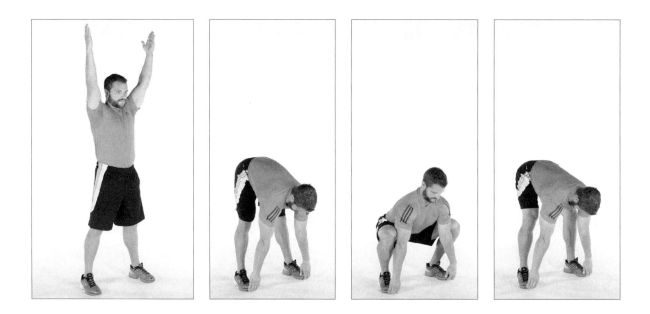

Dynamic Pillar Bridge (TRX)

STEPS

1. In a facedown position, place each foot inside a TRX strap so that the TRX hangs vertically.
2. Supporting your weight on the forearms and feet, tuck your chin so that your head is in line with your body.
3. Keeping your torso stable and your back flat, slowly push your forearms out in

front of you, pushing your feet back behind you as far as you can without losing a stable torso.

4. Reverse the movement pattern to the starting position.
5. Continue for the remainder of the set.

COACHING KEY
Maintain a tight torso and keep your body in a straight line from ear to ankles.

FEEL IT
Working your shoulders and torso.

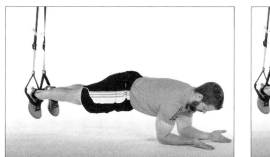
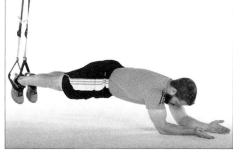

Fencing Stretch

STEPS

1. Standing, step one leg out a quarter turn in line with your opposite heel in about a 3-foot stance.
2. Load the back leg, sitting back in a squat with the front leg straight.
3. Initiating with your pelvis, rotate toward the front leg, spinning on your back foot, bringing your knee underneath you, wrapping your pelvis all the way around.
4. Reverse the motion, again leading with your pelvis.
5. Repeat the movement, focusing on the movement of your pelvis around the head of the femur in the hip socket.

COACHING KEY
Make sure you let your back foot move, so as not to torque your front knee.

FEEL IT
Stretching around your hip, groin, and hip flexors.

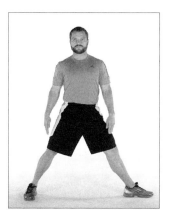
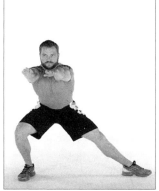
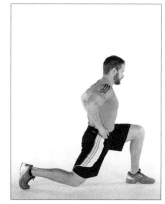

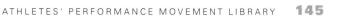

Hip Internal Rotation—Sidelying with Abduction

COACHING KEY

Keep your stomach tight and hamstrings relaxed, and initiate the movement from the inside of your hip.

FEEL IT

Stretching your hips.

STEPS

1. Lie on your side with your hips and knees bent 90 degrees
2. Keeping your knee stationary, rotate your top leg into the air while your top heel remains in contact with your bottom heel.
3. Rotate your heel back to the starting position.
4. Complete the set on one side before repeating on the other side.

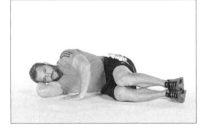
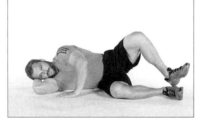
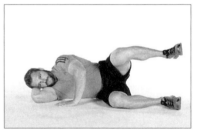

Lateral Line Stretch—Standing

COACHING KEY

Keep your ribs in line with your pelvis. Avoid rotating your torso, as if you are bending sideways between two panes of glass.

FEEL IT

Stretching the sides of your torso.

STEPS

1. Stand tall with a miniband looped around your wrists and your arms straight overhead, pulled slightly apart to create tension in the band.
2. Keeping your torso long and maintaining tension on the band, inhale, and then exhale as you bend at the hip laterally.
3. While maintaining the side-bend, feel your opposite side ribs expand as you breathe.
4. Exhale as you return to the starting position.
5. Repeat the movement in the opposite direction.
6. Continue alternating to complete the set.

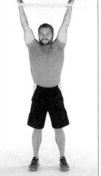
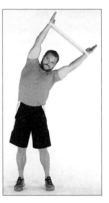

Lateral Pillar Bridge to Row with Hip Flexion

1. Attach a handle to the low pulley of a cable machine. Lie on your side with your chest facing the machine, forearm on the ground under your shoulder, feet stacked, and your top arm holding the handle slightly farther than arm's length.
2. Push your hips off the floor to create a straight line from ankle to shoulder.
3. Pull the handle into your torso as you drive the knee of your top leg forward.
4. Straighten your arm back out in front of you as you return your leg to the starting position.
5. Complete the set on one side before switching sides and repeating with the opposite arm and leg.

COACHING KEY

Keep your torso and hips stable; do not let them sag or move back and forth.

FEEL IT

Working your torso, shoulders, and upper back.

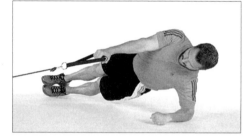
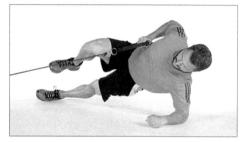

Pillar Bridge—Dynamic Alternating (Arms in TRX)

STEPS

1. In a facedown position, place each forearm inside a TRX strap so that the TRX hangs vertically.
2. Keeping your body in a straight line, reach one arm forward as you keep the other arm stationary.
3. Alternate arms for the prescribed number of repetitions for the remainder of the set.

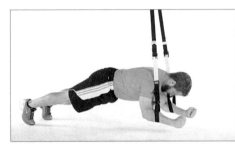 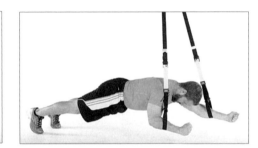

Pillar Bridge—Row to Tricep Extension (Cable)

STEPS

1. Lie facedown in a modified push-up position, with your forearms resting on the floor, supporting your weight on your forearms, facing a cable machine, holding a handle in one hand.
2. Keeping your body straight from ears to ankles, reach the arm holding the handle forward as far as you can.
3. In one continuous motion, pull the handle to your shoulder and then to your hip by extending your elbow.

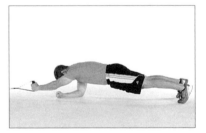

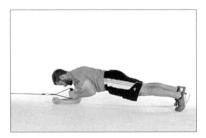

4. Reverse the movement pattern to return to the starting position.
5. Complete the set on one side before repeating with the opposite arm.

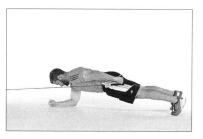

Prone Breathing (Stability Ball)

STEPS

1. Lie facedown with your chest on a large stability ball, completely relaxed, letting your head and arms hang loose.
2. Exhale long and completely, feeling your spine flex over the ball.
3. Take a full, relaxed deep breath.
4. Continue for the full set.

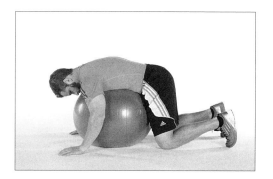

COACHING KEY
Move where the stretch is felt by changing what part of your spine is at the top of the curve of the ball.

FEEL IT
Stretching the back of your torso.

Prone Knee Tuck (TRX)

STEPS

1. Start in the classic push-up position with your hands beneath your shoulders and each foot inside a TRX strap so that the TRX hangs vertically.
2. Keeping your torso stable, pull your knees toward your chest.
3. Reverse the pattern back to the starting position.
4. Continue for the remainder of the set.

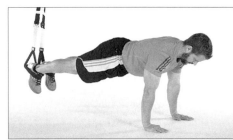
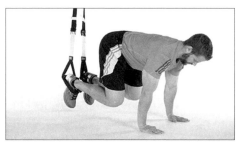

Quadruped Rocking

STEPS

1. Start on all fours with your hands under your shoulders and knees under your hips.
2. Draw your belly button in toward your spine while maintaining a natural curve in your lower back.
3. Move your hips backward until you feel a compression in your hips.
4. Return to the starting position.
5. Continue for the full set.

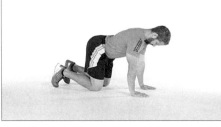
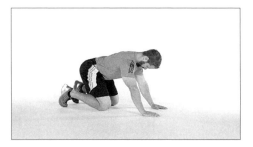

Quadruped Rocking—Wide

1. Start on all fours with your hands under your shoulders and knees wider than hip-width apart.
2. Draw your belly button in toward your spine while maintaining a natural curve in your lower back.
3. Move your hips backward until you feel your pelvis rotate.
4. Return to the starting position.
5. Continue for the full set.

COACHING KEY
Draw your belly button in without losing the curve in your back or feeling your rib cage expand. Think about holding your pelvis still throughout the range of motion.

FEEL IT
Compressing your hips and working your lower back.

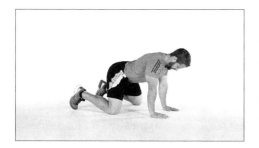
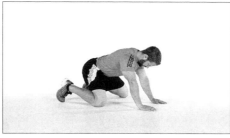

Quadruped Thoracic Spine Rotation—1 Leg Abduction on Wall

COACHING TIP

Reach long through your heel, pushing it into the wall as your trunk rotates to both sides. Keep your hips over your knee throughout the movement.

FEEL IT

Working the mobility of your shoulders, torso, and inner thighs.

STEPS

1. Start on all fours, parallel to a wall with your hands under your shoulders, your outside knee under your hips, and your inside leg straight out to the side with your foot flat against the base of the wall.

2. Lift your head and spine through your shoulder blades toward the ceiling, creating a long line from the crown of your head to your tailbone.

3. Reach your inside arm through the space between your opposite hand and knee as far as you can, rotating your chest away from the wall and bending your outside elbow to assist the stretch.

4. Rotate your torso back through the starting position to point your chest toward the wall and your arm to the sky.

5. Rotate your torso back to the starting position.

6. Reach your outside arm through the space between your opposite hand and knee as far as you can, rotating your chest away from the wall and bending your outside elbow to assist the stretch.

7. Rotate your torso back through the starting position to point your chest away from the wall with your hand on your chest.

8. Complete the set on one side, turn around, and repeat with your opposite leg against the wall.

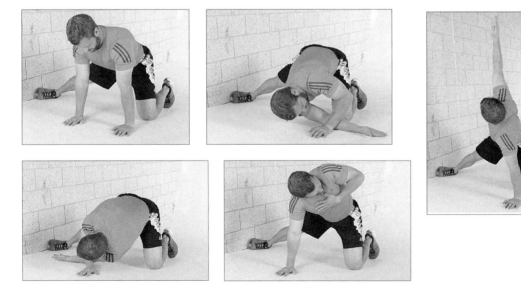

Quadruped Thoracic Spine Rotation—1 Leg Extended on Wall

1. Start on all fours, facing away from a wall with your hands under your shoulders, one knee under your hip, and the other straight back with your foot flat against the wall.
2. Lift your head and spine through your shoulder blades toward the ceiling, creating a long line from the crown of your head to your tailbone.
3. Reach your same-side arm of your bent leg through the space between your opposite hand and knee as far as you can, rotating your chest and bending your outside elbow to assist the stretch.
4. Rotate your torso back through the starting position to point your chest to the opposite side while keeping your hand on your chest.
5. Rotate your torso back to the starting position.
6. Complete the set on one side, switch legs, and repeat.

COACHING TIP
Reach long through your heel, pushing it into the wall as your trunk rotates to both sides. Keep your hips over your knee throughout the movement.

FEEL IT
Working the mobility of your shoulders, torso, and hips.

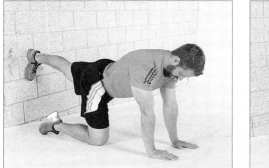
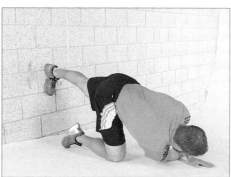
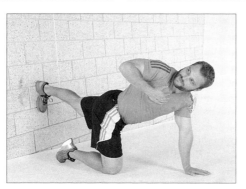

Quadruped Weight Shift

COACHING KEY
Do not lock your elbows as you shift your weight.

FEEL IT
Working your hips, shoulders, and torso.

STEPS

1. Start on all fours with your arms straight under your shoulders, knees under your hips, and shoulders pushed away from the floor.
2. Inhale and shift to one side of your body, feeling your shoulder blade, torso, and hip accept more weight.
3. Exhale and return to the starting position.
4. Repeat the move, shifting your weight to the opposite side.
5. Exhale and return to the starting position.
6. Continue alternating to complete the set.

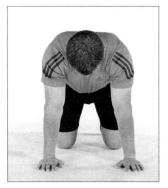
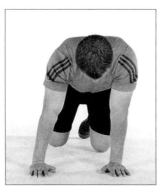
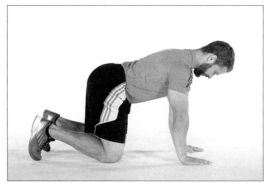

Segmental Glute Bridge

STEPS

1. Lie on your back with your hips and knees bent.
2. Exhale and roll your pelvis to lift just your glutes off the ground.
3. Slowly peel your spine off the floor, one segment of your spine at a time, until you create a straight line from your shoulders to your knees.
4. Pause at the top of your range of motion and take a small inhale breath.
5. Exhale and reverse the movement pattern, slowly rolling each segment of your spine back to the starting position.
6. Continue for the full set.

COACHING KEY

Keep your neck and shoulders relaxed. Visualize picking your spine off the floor like a beaded necklace. Breathe more than once if needed, moving on the exhale and pausing on the inhale.

FEEL IT

Working your abs, glutes, hamstrings, and spine.

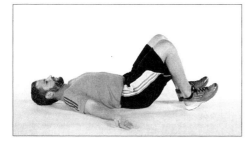
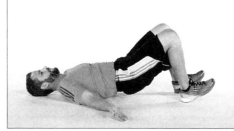
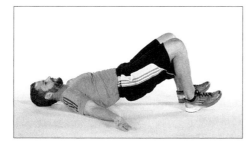
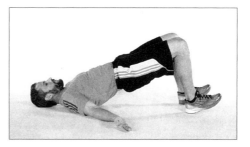

Segmental Glute Bridge—
Lateral Shift

COACHING KEY

Keep your neck and shoulders relaxed and your pelvis level throughout the movement.

FEEL IT

Working your abs, glutes, hamstrings, and spine.

STEPS

1. Lie on your back with your hips and knees bent.
2. Exhale and roll your pelvis to lift just your glutes off the ground.
3. Slowly peel your spine off the floor, one segment of your spine at a time, until you create a straight line from your shoulders to your knees.
4. Pause at the top of your range of motion and take a small inhale breath.
5. Shift your hips to one side without dropping or rotating your pelvis.
6. Pause, then shift your pelvis to the opposite side.
7. Exhale and reverse the movement pattern, slowly rolling each segment of your spine back to the starting position.
8. Continue for the full set.

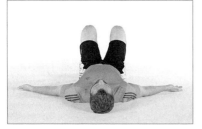 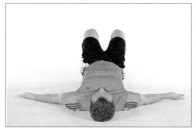 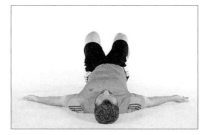

Sidelying Quad/Hip Flexor Stretch with Rotation

STEPS

1. Lie on your side with both knees pulled toward your chest, holding your top ankle with your top hand.
2. Contract your top glute and pull your top leg back until you feel a stretch in the front of your thigh.
3. Inhale and hold the stretch for 2 seconds.
4. Still holding your ankle, exhale as you rotate your torso to the ground so that your chest points up.
5. Inhale and hold the stretch for 2 seconds.
6. Exhale and return to the starting position.
7. Complete the set on one side before repeating on the opposite leg.

COACHING KEY

Contract the glute of your top leg and keep your hips perpendicular to the floor throughout the stretch.

FEEL IT

Stretching the quadriceps and hip flexor of your top leg.

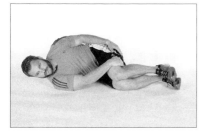
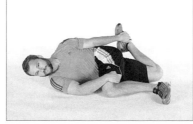
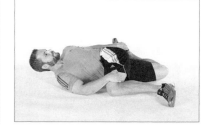

Standing Toe Taps

1. Stand with your legs hip-width apart and shift your weight over the middle of your arches.
2. Without shifting your body weight, lift just your toes off the ground.
3. Lay down each toe one at a time, starting at the pinkie and working your way in.
4. Complete the set in this direction and then repeat, starting with your big toe and working your way out.

COACHING KEY
Think about spreading your toes apart as you lift and lower them.

FEEL IT
Working the small muscles in the bottom of your feet.

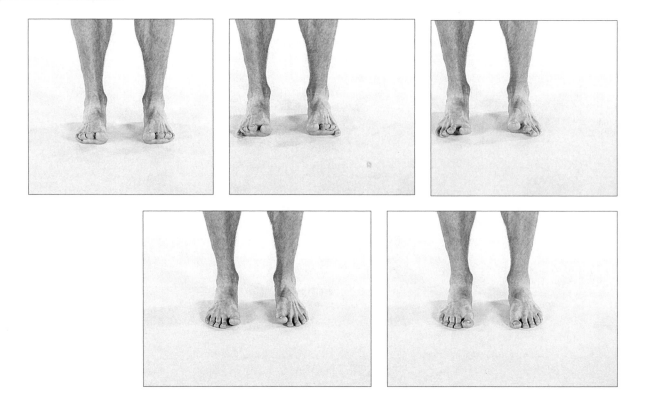

Step to Inverted Hamstring Stretch

1. Stand tall with your chest up.
2. Slowly lean forward, bending only at your ankles until you have to step forward with one foot to catch your balance.
3. In one continuous motion, step forward to catch your balance and bend forward at the waist as your back leg lifts straight behind you.
4. When you feel a stretch in the back of your thigh, return to the starting position by contracting the glute and hamstring of your planted leg.
5. Repeat the movement, catching yourself with your opposite foot.
6. Continue alternating to complete the set.

COACHING KEY

Keep your back flat. Someone should be able to place a broomstick snugly across your back at the bottom of the move.

FEEL IT

Challenging your balance, stretching your hamstrings, and working your ankles.

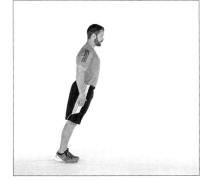
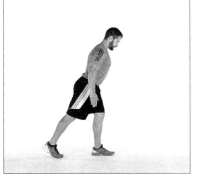
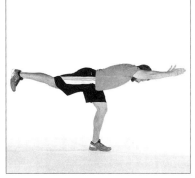

Straight Leg Lowering

STEPS

1. Lie flat on your back with your arms at your sides and both legs straight up in the air over your hips.
2. Keeping one leg straight, slowly lower the other leg down along an arc to just above the floor.
3. Return to the starting position and repeat the move with your opposite leg.
4. Continue alternating to complete the set.

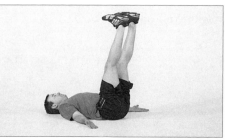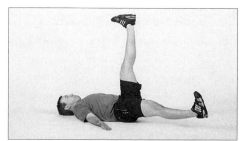

Supine Active Hip Rotator Stretch

STEPS

1. Lie faceup with your hips and knees bent, heels on the ground and toes off the ground.
2. Without letting your pelvis rotate, lift one leg up and cross it over the opposite knee at the ankle.
3. Inhale and dorsiflex (bend up) your ankle.
4. Exhale and push your knee away from your torso.
5. Inhale and release the stretch.
6. Complete the set on one side before repeating on the opposite leg.

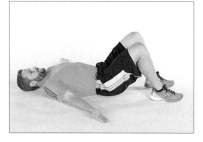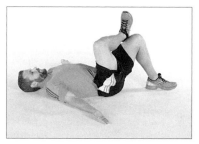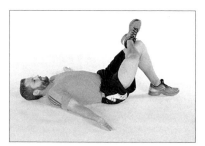

Supine Fallout at 90-Degree
Hip Flexion with Front Line Connection

STEPS

1. Lie on your back with your hips and knees bent, hip-width apart, with your heels on the ground.
2. Inhale as you lift one leg up so that your hip and knee are bent at 90 degrees. Exhale.
3. Inhale as you lift the other leg to the same position. Exhale.
4. Plantarflex (point) one ankle and Dorsiflex (pull up) the opposite ankle.
5. Inhale as you let the dorsiflexed ankle leg fall to the side as far as you can without moving your torso or pelvis.
6. Exhale, bring the leg back, and repeat the breathing and leg lowering pattern.
7. Complete the set on one side before repeating with the other leg.

COACHING KEY

Keep the range of motion of the fallout controlled so that your pelvis and low back do not move.

FEEL IT

Working your abs and hips.

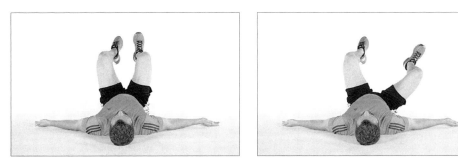

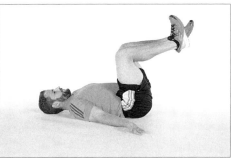

Toe Finger Weave—Circles

STEPS

1. Sit on the floor with one ankle crossed over your opposite thigh.
2. Use one hand to support your weight and the other to weave your fingers between your toes.
3. Relax your foot and ankle and use your hand to rotate your foot in circles.
4. Circle clockwise for the prescribed number of repetitions and then repeat counterclockwise.
5. Complete the set on one side before repeating on the other side.

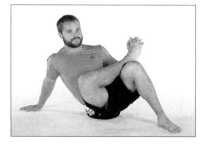
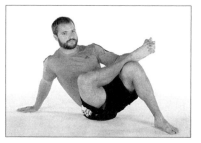
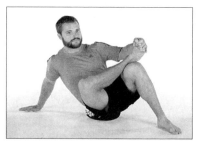

Toe Wall Walks

1. Lie faceup with your knees and hips bent to 90 degrees each, your feet flat against a wall, and your arms by your sides.
2. While maintaining contact with the wall, walk your feet as far as you can up the wall by curling your toes and pulling your feet up.
3. At the end of your range of motion, walk your feet back down the wall by curling your toes and pushing your feet down.
4. Continue for the full set.

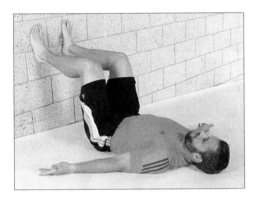
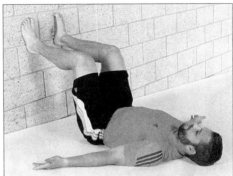
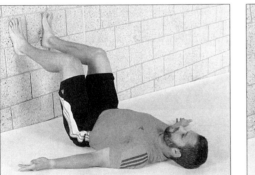
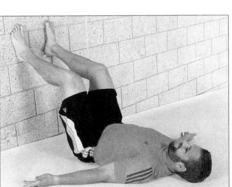

COACHING KEY

Keep your toes pointed straight to the ceiling and your torso stable throughout the move.

FEEL IT

Working the small muscles of your foot and stretching the front of your ankle.

Toe Waves

COACHING KEY
Keep your foot and
ankle pointed
straight ahead.

FEEL IT
Stretching the
small muscles
in the bottom of
your feet.

STEPS

1. Sit with shoes off and your feet relaxed on the ground.
2. Initiate the movement at your toes by extending them up and then bending your ankle up into dorsiflexion.
3. Reverse the movement pattern, starting by bending your ankle down into plantarflexion and then flexing your toes down.
4. Continue repeating this wave motion for the remainder of the set.

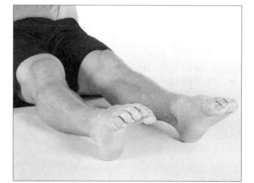
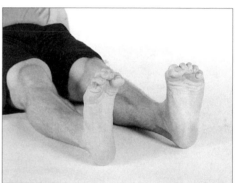
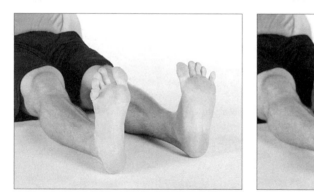

2-Inch Runs—in Place

STEPS

1. Stand in an athletic base position with your knees slightly bent, hips back, and arms bent slightly throughout the move.
2. Run in place by moving your feet two inches up and down, with each step as quick as possible, allowing your arms to move rhythmically.
3. Continue for the prescribed amount of time.

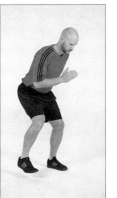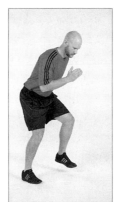

COACHING KEY
Try to make your feet "pop" rather than "scuff" as you run.

FEEL IT
Working your hips, knees, and ankles and challenging your coordination.

Base Rotations

STEPS

1. Stand in an athletic base position with your knees slightly bent and hips back.
2. Keeping your chest facing straight ahead, rapidly jump slightly off the floor and rotate your hips to the right as you move your arms left.
3. Land and immediately jump back to your left, moving your arms right.
4. Continue for the prescribed amount of time.

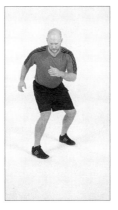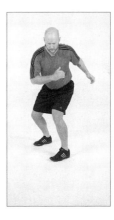

COACHING KEY
Use your arms to counterbalance the movement and focus on swiveling your hips, not your shoulders and torso.

FEEL IT
Working your hips, knees, and ankles and challenging your coordination.

Crossover Skip

COACHING KEY

Keep your chest pointed forward and feel your hips swivel as you drive your knee across your body and return it back to the base position.

FEEL IT

Working your entire body.

STEPS

1. Stand tall with your arms at your sides.
2. Drive one knee up and across your body.
3. Drive your lifted leg down to the ground on the outside of your other foot as you create a double foot contact.
4. Use the force of the contact to square your hips to face forward and immediately repeat this pattern to continue moving laterally.
5. Complete the set for the prescribed number of repetitions on one side before repeating in the opposite direction.

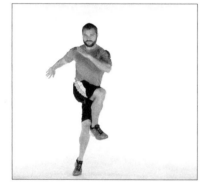
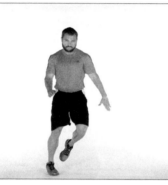
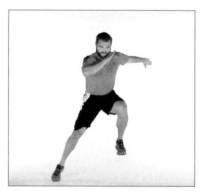

Drop Lunge

STEPS

1. Stand tall with your arms at your sides.
2. Reach one foot back behind and across your other foot.
3. Square your hips back to the starting position, and then sit back and down into a squat.
4. Push through your hip to stand up.
5. Complete the set on one side before repeating on the other side.

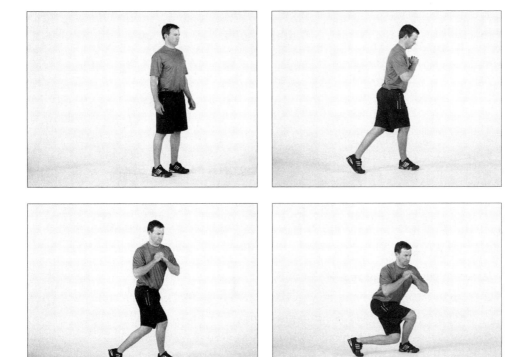

Dropstep Skip

STEPS

1. Stand tall with your feet hip-width apart, knees slightly bent, hips back, and elbows bent to 90 degrees.
2. Lift one knee in the air as you open up your hips, countering the movement by swinging your opposite arm forward and same-side arm back.
3. Plant your foot behind you and generate a double foot contact before you lift your opposite leg.
4. Continue this skipping pattern to complete the set.

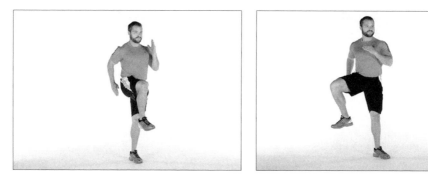

Dropstep Squat

STEPS

1. Stand tall with your feet together.
2. Step to the side and behind you with one foot so that your hips open and your feet point out in a classic sumo position.
3. Lower your hips and squat down into a comfortable stretch.
4. Stand up and return to the starting position.
5. Complete the set on one side before repeating with the opposite leg.

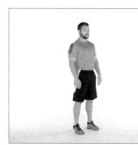 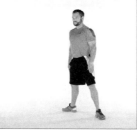 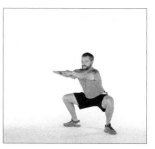

Handwalk

STEPS

1. Stand with your legs straight and your hands on the ground in front of you.
2. Keeping your legs straight and stomach tight, walk your hands forward to a push-up position.
3. Still keeping your legs straight, walk your feet back up to your hands.
4. When a stretch is felt, walk your hands back out to a push-up position.
5. Continue to complete the set.

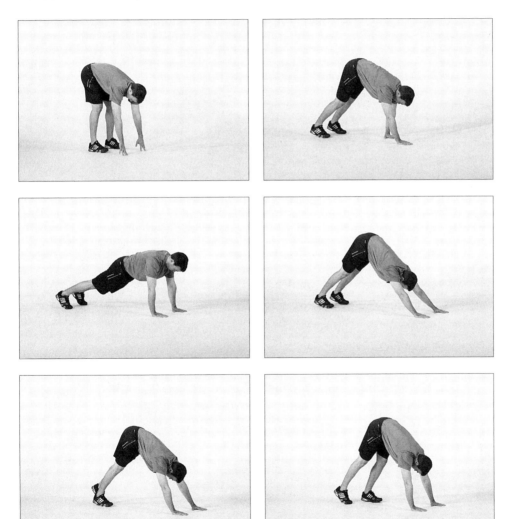

Inverted Hamstring

1. Stand tall on one leg with your chest up, your shoulder blades back and down, and a stretch band looped around your shoulder and foot that is in the air.
2. Raise your arms out to your sides with your thumbs up.
3. Keeping a straight line between your ear and ankle, bend forward at the waist and lift your other leg straight behind you.
4. When you feel a stretch in the back of your thigh, return to the starting position by contracting the glute and hamstring of your planted leg.
5. Complete the set on one side before repeating with the opposite leg.

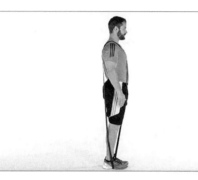
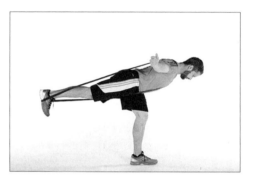

Knee Hug

STEPS

1. Stand tall with your arms at your sides.
2. Lift one foot off the ground and squat back and down a few inches with the other leg.
3. Contracting the glute of your standing leg, grab below your lifted knee with your hands and pull your knee to your chest while straightening your other leg. Hold for 1 to 2 seconds.
4. Relax and return to the starting position.
5. Repeat the movement with your other leg.
6. Continue alternating to complete the set.

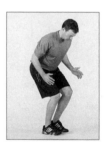
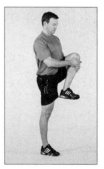

Lateral Lunge

1. Step to one side and lower your hips to the floor by squatting back and down with the stepping leg, keeping the other leg straight.
2. Return to the starting position by pushing up with your bent leg.
3. Switch directions and repeat the movement.
4. Continue alternating to complete the set.

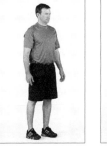 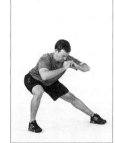

COACHING KEY
Keep your chest up and your back flat.

FEEL IT
Working your glutes, hamstrings, and quads and stretching the inner thigh of the straight leg.

Leg Cradle

STEPS

1. Stand with your back straight, knees unlocked, and arms at your sides.
2. Lift one foot off the ground and squat back and down a few inches with the other leg.
3. Contracting the glute of your standing leg, grab below your lifted knee with your same-side hand and under your ankle with your other hand.
4. Extend your standing leg as you pull your opposite knee up and across your body until you feel a gentle stretch in the outside of your hip.
5. Return to the starting position and repeat with your other leg.
6. Continue alternating to complete the set.

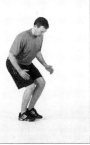 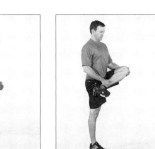

COACHING KEY
Focus on standing tall, keeping your chest up throughout the move.

FEEL IT
Stretching the outside of your hip.

Miniband Walking—Lateral, Bent Knee

STEPS

1. Start in a squat position with your back flat, hips back, and a miniband around your knees.
2. Taking small steps no more than 6 inches apart, walk sideways by pushing off of your trailing leg.
3. Continue laterally for the prescribed number of steps, then reverse directions using the same technique for the prescribed number of steps.

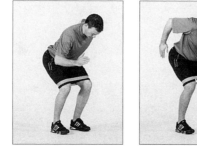 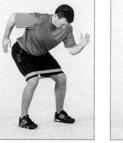 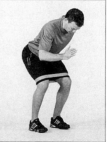

Miniband Walking—Linear, Bent Knee

STEPS

1. Start in a squat position with your back flat, hips back, and a miniband around your ankles.
2. Taking small steps, walk forward, keeping your feet in line with your hips.
3. Continue forward for the prescribed number of steps, then walk backward using the same technique for the prescribed number of steps.

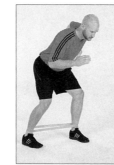 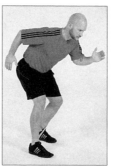 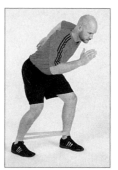

Pillar March—Lateral

1. Stand tall with your arms at your sides and elbows bent to 90 degrees.
2. Lift one knee up while you bring the opposite arm forward and the same-side elbow back.
3. Step to the side by driving your foot down to the ground, lifting your opposite knee and exchanging arm positions.
4. Continue marching laterally for the prescribed number of steps.
5. Repeat the movement in the opposite direction.

COACHING KEY
Fully extend and push off with your trailing leg.

FEEL IT
Working your entire body.

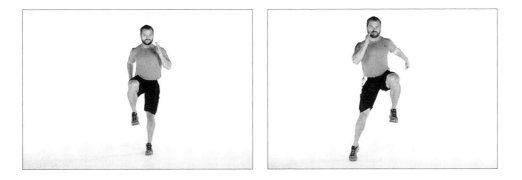

Pillar March—Linear

STEPS

1. Stand with your arms at your sides and your elbows bent 90 degrees.
2. Lift one knee up while you bring the opposite arm forward and the same-side elbow back.
3. March forward by driving your foot down to the ground, lifting your opposite knee and exchanging arm positions.
4. Continue the movement for the prescribed number of steps.

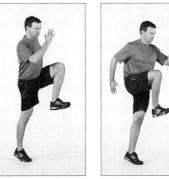

COACHING KEY
Initiate the movement from your glutes, and think about pushing your trailing foot through the ground as you fully extend your hips.

FEEL IT
Working your entire body.

Pillar Skip—Lateral

COACHING KEY
Fully extend and push off with your trailing leg.

FEEL IT
Working your entire body.

STEPS

1. Stand tall with your arms at your sides and elbows bent to 90 degrees.
2. Lift one knee up while you bring the opposite arm forward and the same-side elbow back.
3. Skip to the side by driving your foot down to the ground, generating a double foot contact, as your opposite foot and knee lift and your arms exchange positions.
4. Continue laterally in the same direction by repeating the movement with the opposite leg.
5. Continue this skipping pattern for the prescribed number of skips on each side.
6. Repeat the movement in the opposite direction.

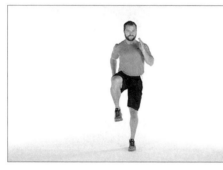

Pillar Skip—Linear

COACHING KEY
Fully extend and push off with your trailing leg.

FEEL IT
Working your entire body.

STEPS

1. Stand tall with your arms at your sides and elbows bent to 90 degrees.
2. Lift one knee up while you bring the opposite arm forward and the same-side elbow back.

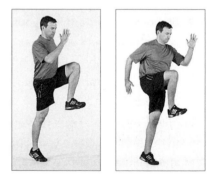

3. Skip forward by driving your foot down to the ground, generating a double foot contact, as your opposite foot and knee lift and your arms exchange positions.
4. Continue to skip forward by repeating the movement with the opposite leg.
5. Continue alternating for the prescribed number of steps to complete the set.

Reverse Lunge—Forearm to Instep with Rotation

STEPS

1. Stand tall with your arms at your sides.
2. Step backward into a lunge with your right foot.
3. Place your right hand on the ground and your left elbow to the inside of your left foot. Hold this stretch for 1 to 2 seconds.
4. Rotate your left arm and chest to the sky. Hold again for 1 to 2 seconds.
5. Bring your left arm down and reach it across under your torso to the opposite side.
6. Return to standing, repeat the movement on the opposite side and repeat for the prescribed number of repetitions.

COACHING KEY

As you lunge, contract the glute of your back leg to help stretch the front of your hip.

FEEL IT

Stretching your groin, hip flexor of your back leg, and glute and hamstrings of your front leg.

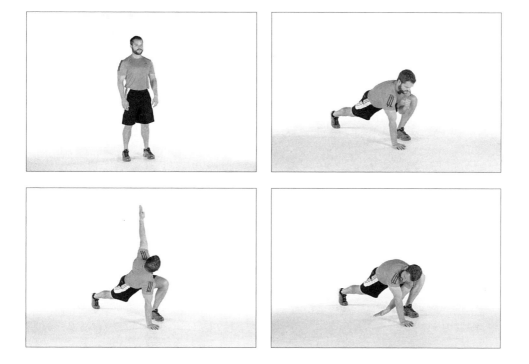

Tinioca

COACHING KEY
Your steps should be short and quick. Keep your shoulders facing forward while rotating your hips as quickly as possible.

FEEL IT
Working your entire body.

STEPS

1. Stand with your feet shoulder-width apart and your arms out to your sides at shoulder level.
2. Cross your right leg in front of your left leg as you rotate your hips and arms in opposite directions and begin moving left.
3. Move your left leg and hips back to the base position while pushing off your right leg and rotating your arms in the opposite direction.
4. Bring your right leg behind your left leg, rotate your hips and arms in opposite directions, and continue moving left.
5. Continue this pattern to complete the set on one side before repeating in the opposite direction.

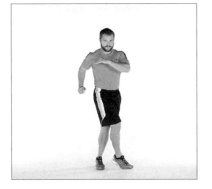
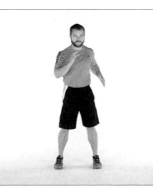
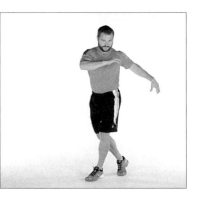

Box Jump

STEPS

1. Stand with your feet slightly wider than shoulder-width apart. This exercise can also be done wearing a weight vest.

2. Keeping your chest up, squat down and immediately jump vertically onto a box, extending through your hips and pulling your toes toward your shins in midair.

3. Land softly in a squat position.

4. Stand and reset to the starting position.

5. Continue for the full set.

COACHING KEY
Do not pause at the bottom of the movement.

FEEL IT
Working your hips, knees, and ankles.

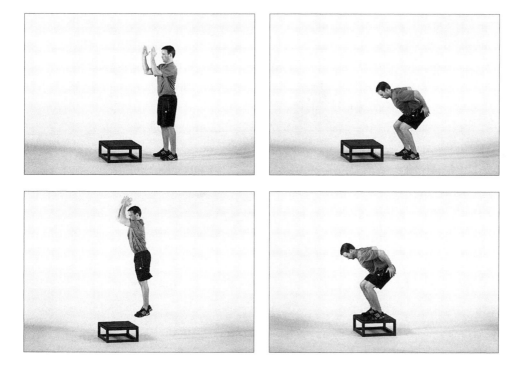

Drop Squat—2 Feet to 1 Foot

COACHING KEY
Move with speed, but make sure to stick your landing.

FEEL IT
Working your hips and legs.

STEPS

1. Stand tall with your feet wider than shoulder-width apart and your arms bent upward at 90 degrees in front of you.
2. Lift your feet off the ground and throw your arms behind you as you sit back and down and land on one leg in a partial squat.
3. Stand and repeat the movement, landing on the opposite leg.
4. Continue alternating to complete the set.

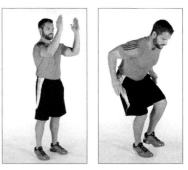

Horizontal Jump

COACHING KEY
Use your arms to help you drive up and out during your jump.

FEEL IT
Working your entire body.

STEPS

1. Stand tall with your arms bent 90 degrees and your forearms pointed up.
2. Drive elbows back as you drop into a squat by bending your knees and pushing your hips back.
3. Immediately push the ground away from you, jumping up and out as far as you can.
4. Land softly in a squat position and return to the start position.
5. Continue for the full set.

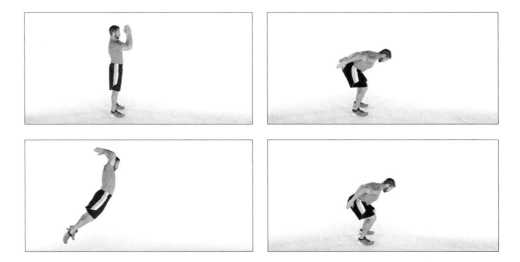

Lateral Bound—Continuous

1. Stand with your hips and knees slightly bent.
2. Generating force with your arms, bound to one side by extending the hip, knee, and ankle of one leg.
3. Land on the opposite leg and, without pausing, bound in the opposite direction.
4. Continue bounding to complete the set.

COACHING KEY

Try to jump as high and far as possible while landing balanced.

FEEL IT

Working your hips and legs.

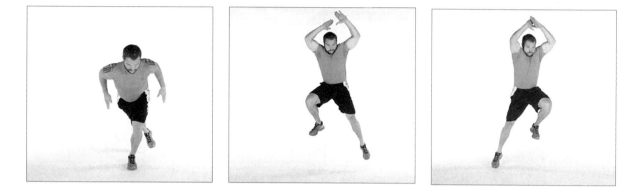

Lateral Bound—Quick and Stabilize

COACHING KEY

Try to jump as high and far as possible while landing balanced.

FEEL IT

Working your hips and legs.

STEPS

1. Stand with your hips and knees slightly bent. This exercise can also be done wearing a weight vest.
2. Generating force with your arms, bound to one side by extending the hip, knee, and ankle of one leg.
3. Land on the opposite leg and, without pausing, bound in the opposite direction.
4. Land softly and hold for 3 seconds.
5. Continue alternating to complete the set.

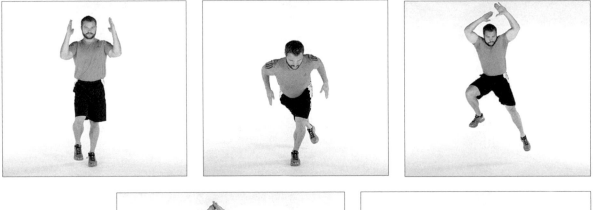

Lateral Bound—Stabilize

1. Stand with your hips and knees slightly bent with a miniband around your thighs just above your knees. This exercise can also be done wearing a weight vest.
2. Generating force with your arms, bound to one side by extending the hip, knee, and ankle of one leg.
3. Land softly on your opposite leg by absorbing the impact with your hip and hold for 3 seconds.
4. Stand and repeat the movement in the opposite direction, bounding off your opposite leg.
5. Continue alternating to complete the set.

COACHING KEY

Focus on jumping for maximum height and distance, and then stick the landing.

FEEL IT

Working your hips and legs.

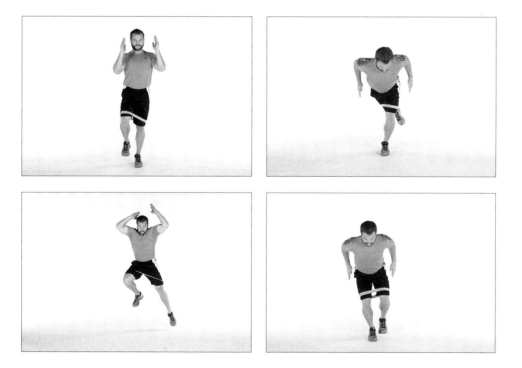

Lateral Hurdle Hop—Continuous

COACHING KEY

Land softly by absorbing the impact with your hips. Anticipate the ground to minimize contact time.

FEEL IT

Working your hips and legs.

STEPS

1. Stand with your side to a line of hurdles, balancing on your inside leg with your arms bent 90 degrees. This exercise can also be done wearing a weight vest.
2. Propelling yourself with your arms and hips, hop laterally over the line of hurdles without pausing when you land.
3. At the end of the hurdles, stick the landing, switch legs, and repeat the movement in the opposite direction.
4. Continue alternating to complete the set.

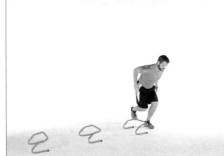
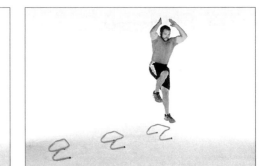
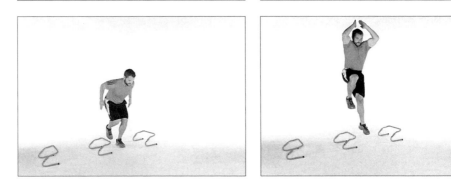

Lateral Hurdle Hop—Double Contact to Stabilize

1. Stand with your side to a line of hurdles, balancing on your inside leg with your arms bent 90 degrees. This exercise can also be done wearing a weight vest.
2. Propelling yourself with your arms and hips, bounce on your takeoff foot to preload, and then hop laterally over the first hurdle.
3. Absorb the impact through your hip to land softly and stabilize for 1 to 2 seconds.
4. Continue over the remaining hurdles.
5. At the end of the hurdles, stick the landing, switch legs, and repeat the movement in the opposite direction.
6. Continue alternating to complete the set.

COACHING KEY
Fully extend your hip on each hop.

FEEL IT
Working your hips and legs.

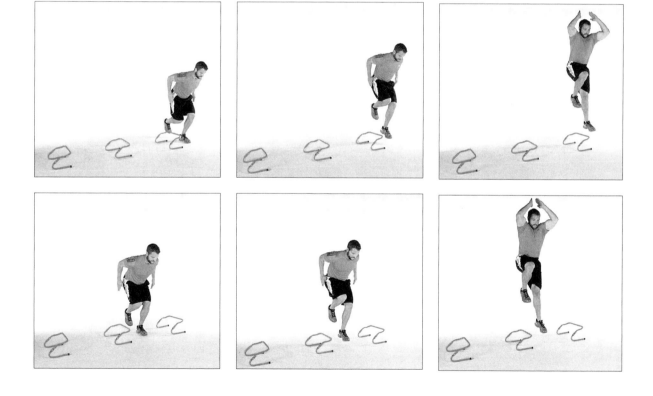

Linear Bound—Quick and Stabilize

COACHING KEY

Bound as high and far as possible while focusing on sticking the landing.

FEEL IT

Working your hips and legs.

STEPS

1. Stand tall on one leg with your feet hip-width apart and your elbows bent 90 degrees.
2. Dip down slightly at the hip and knee and pull your elbows behind you.
3. Immediately bound forward, generating force by driving your arms toward the sky and pushing off the ground.
4. Land on your opposite leg and, without pausing, bound forward with this leg.
5. Land softly on your opposite leg by absorbing the impact with your hip. Hold for 2 to 3 seconds, and then stand.
6. Repeat the movement on the opposite leg.
7. Continue alternating to complete the set.

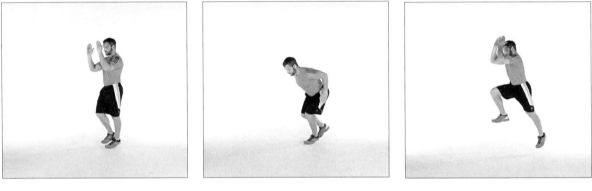

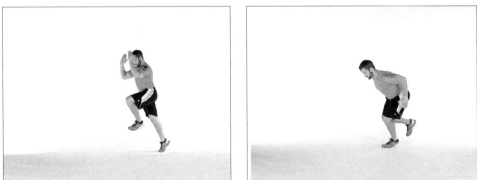

Linear Hurdle Hop—Continuous

1. Stand in front of a line of hurdles, balancing on one leg with your elbows bent 90 degrees. This exercise can also be done wearing a weight vest.
2. Drive your elbows back as you dip your hips back and down.
3. Using your arms and hips to generate force, hop over the first hurdle.
4. Land on the same leg, anticipating the ground to minimize contact time and, without pausing, hop over the next hurdle.
5. Continue over the remaining hurdles, initiating each hop by sitting back and down with your hips.
6. Switch legs and repeat the movement in the opposite direction.

COACHING KEY

Land softly and absorb the impact through your hip without letting your knee collapse to the inside.

FEEL IT

Working your hips and legs.

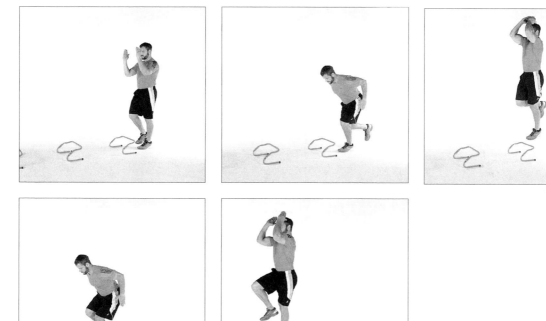

Linear Hurdle Hop—Countermovement

COACHING KEY

Land softly and absorb the impact through your hip without letting your knee collapse to the inside.

FEEL IT

Working your hips and legs.

STEPS

1. Stand in front of a line of hurdles, balancing on one leg with your elbows bent 90 degrees. This exercise can also be done wearing a weight vest.
2. Drive your elbows back as you dip your hips back and down.
3. Immediately hop over the first hurdle, using your arms and hips to generate force.
4. Stabilize upon landing and return to a standing position.
5. Continue over the remaining hurdles, initiating each hop by sitting back and down with your hips.
6. Switch legs and repeat the movement in the opposite direction.

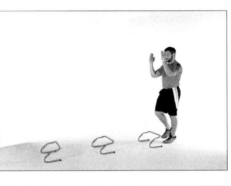
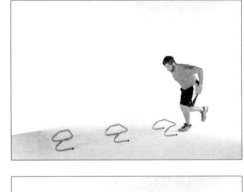
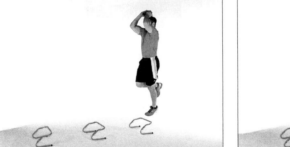
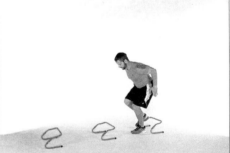

Linear Hurdle Hop—Double Contact to Stabilize

STEPS

1. Stand in front of a line of hurdles, balancing on one leg with your elbows bent 90 degrees. This exercise can also be done wearing a weight vest.
2. Propelling yourself with your arms and hips, bounce on your foot to preload, and then hop over the first hurdle.
3. Absorb the impact through your hip to land softly and stabilize for 1 to 2 seconds.
4. Continue over the remaining hurdles.
5. At the end of the hurdles, stick the landing, switch legs, and repeat the movement.

COACHING KEY
Fully extend your hip on each hop and do not allow your knee to collapse to the inside on takeoff or landing.

FEEL IT
Working your hips and legs.

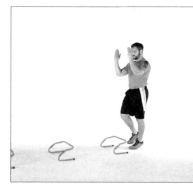
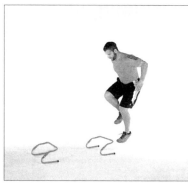
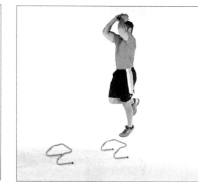
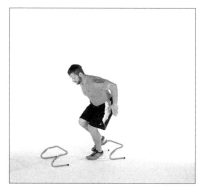
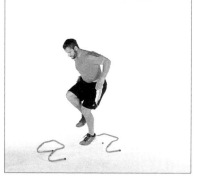

Rotational Bound—90-Degree Quick and Stabilize

COACHING KEY
Do not allow your knee to collapse to the inside during takeoff or landing.

FEEL IT
Working your hips and legs.

STEPS

1. Balance on one leg.
2. Using your hips and arms to generate force, dip your hips and knees down and bound up and to the side, rotating 90 degrees in the air.
3. Land on the opposite leg and, without pausing, bound in the opposite direction.
4. Land softly and hold for 3 seconds.
5. Alternate for prescribed number of repetitions.

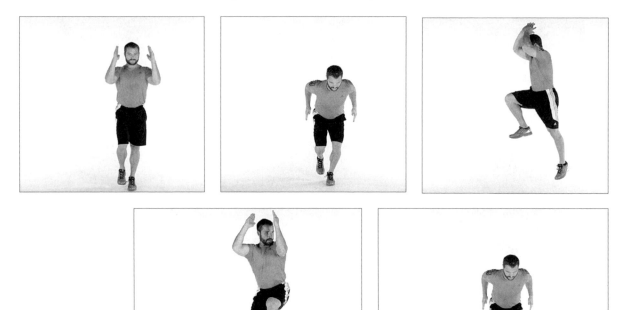

Squat Jump—Countermovement

1. Stand with your feet slightly wider than shoulder-width and your shoulders and elbows flexed to 90 degrees. This exercise can also be done wearing a weight vest.
2. Keeping your chest up, squat down while driving your elbows back behind you and immediately jump vertically, extending through your hips and throwing your elbows forward.
3. Land softly in a squat position.
4. Stand and reset to the starting position.
5. Continue for the full set.

COACHING KEY
Do not pause at the bottom of the movement.

FEEL IT
Working your hips, knees, and ankles.

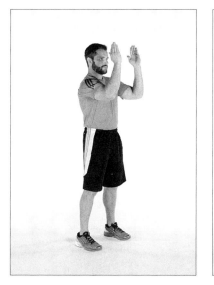
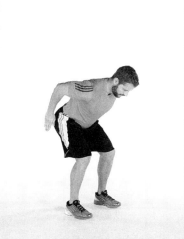
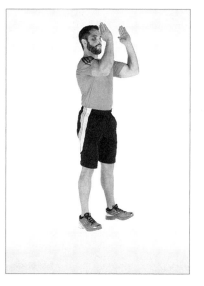

Squat Jump— Non-Countermovement

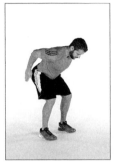
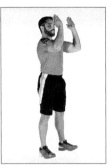

STEPS

1. Stand with your feet slightly wider than shoulder-width apart. This exercise can also be done wearing a weight vest.
2. Sit back and down into a squat and pause with your elbows back behind your body.
3. Jump straight up, pulling your toes toward your shins in midair.
4. Land softly in a squat position and hold for 3 seconds.
5. Continue for the remainder of the set.

Straight-Leg Skip

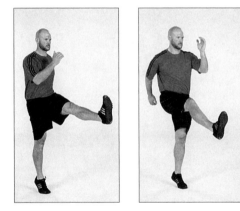

STEPS

1. Stand tall with your arms at your sides.
2. Lift one leg straight in front of your body as your opposite arm swings forward.
3. Use your glutes to pull your heel back down to the ground and generate a double contact with your foot, moving your body forward as the other leg and arm swing forward.
4. Repeat the movement pattern for the full set.

Acceleration Sled Drill—Sprint

STEPS

1. Stand in an athletic base position with your knees and hips slightly bent and your arms bent at your sides, with a sled attached to your waist.
2. Accelerate forward, lifting one knee and the opposite arm while maintaining a forward lean and good posture.
3. Drive your foot down to the ground as the opposite foot and knee lift.
4. Continue alternating to complete the set.

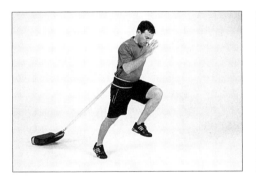 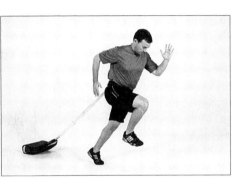

COACHING KEY

Initiate the movement from your glutes. Think about pushing your trailing foot through the ground as you fully extend your hips.

FEEL IT

Working your entire body.

Acceleration Wall Drill— Load and Lift

STEPS

1. Stand leaning forward with your hands on a wall and your ears, shoulders, hips, knees, and ankles in a straight line.
2. Extend one leg straight behind you as you bend your opposite knee and lower your hips back and down.
3. Bring the knee and foot of your back leg toward the wall and hold for 1 to 2 seconds.
4. Continue for the remainder of the set and repeat on the opposite side.

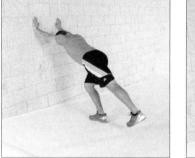 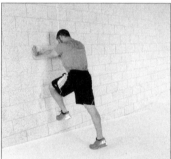

Acceleration Wall Drill— Posture Hold

STEPS

1. Stand leaning forward with your hands on a wall and your ears, shoulders, hips, knees, and ankles in a straight line.
2. Lift one knee and foot toward the wall.
3. Hold this position for the prescribed amount of time.
4. Repeat the movement on your opposite leg.

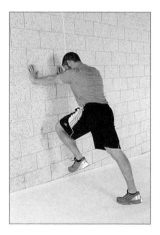

Acceleration Wall Drill— Single Exchange

STEPS
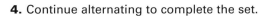

1. Stand leaning forward with your hands on a wall and your ears, shoulders, hips, knees, and ankles in a straight line.
2. Lift one knee and foot toward the wall and pause.
3. Quickly drive the same foot back to the starting position as you lift the other knee toward the wall and then pause.
4. Continue alternating to complete the set.

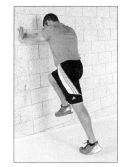

Accelerations

STEPS

1. Stand with your feet hip-width apart in a split stance so one foot is in front of the other.
2. Without stepping backward, accelerate forward by driving out of your front hip, maintaining a forward lean and good posture.
3. Continue to accelerate forward for the prescribed distance.
4. Switch legs and repeat.
5. Continue alternating to complete the set.

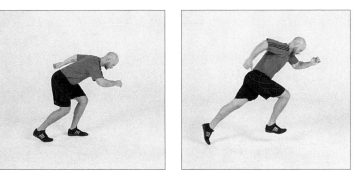

Crossover Drill—Quick and Stabilize

STEPS

1. Place 2 cones about 3 meters apart. Starting at one cone with the other out to your side, stand in an athletic base position with your knees slightly bent, hips back, and arms bent in front of you.
2. Drive one knee up and across your body and plant your foot outside your opposite leg.
3. Snap your hips open to bring the opposite foot back to a base position at the other cone.
4. Immediately reverse direction, repeat the movement, and pause at the starting position.
5. Complete the set on one side before repeating on the opposite side.

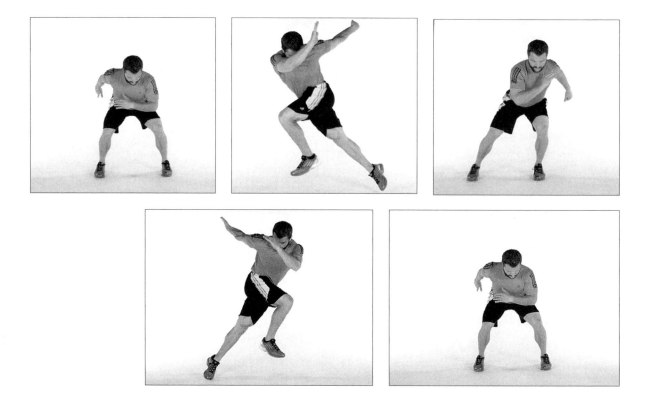

Crossover Drill—
Resisted Continuous

STEPS

1. Stand in an athletic base position with a bungee attached at your waist.
2. With resistance from the bungee, drive your knee up and across your body away from the bungee and plant your foot outside your opposite leg, pushing the ground away from you.
3. Snap your hips open to bring your feet back to the base position.
4. Repeat the movement in the opposite direction to return to the starting position.
5. Complete the set on one side before repeating in the opposite direction.

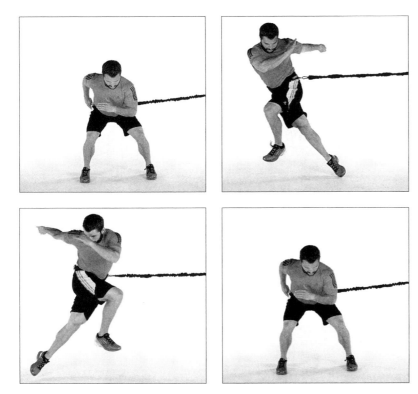

Lateral Shuffle—Continuous

Do not allow your feet to come together. Minimize the amount of time during each change of direction.

FEEL IT
Working your entire body.

STEPS

1. Place 2 cones about 4 yards apart. Starting at one cone with the other out to your side, stand in an athletic base position.
2. Shuffle laterally to the opposite cone, pushing with your outside leg and picking up with your inside foot.
3. Immediately reverse direction.
4. Without pausing, continue to shuffle back and forth for the remainder of the set.

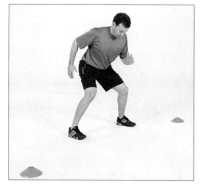 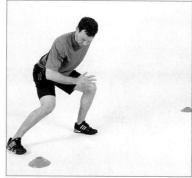 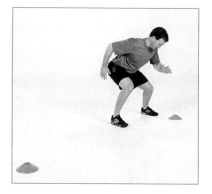

Lateral Shuffle—Quick and Stabilize

STEPS

1. Place 2 cones about 4 yards apart. Starting at one cone with the other out to your side, stand in an athletic base position.
2. Shuffle laterally to the opposite cone, pushing with your outside leg and picking up with your inside foot.
3. Immediately reverse direction, shuffle back to the starting position, and pause for 3 seconds.
4. Complete the set on one side before repeating in the opposite direction.

COACHING KEY
Do not allow your feet to come together. Minimize the amount of time during the change of direction.

FEEL IT
Working your entire body.

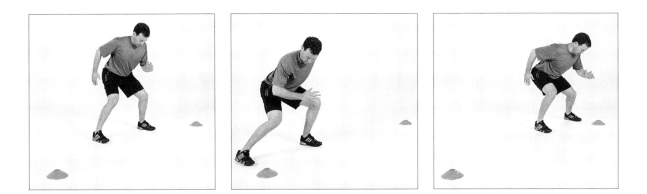

Lateral Shuffle—Resisted Continuous

COACHING KEY

Do not allow your feet to come together. Minimize the amount of time during each change of direction.

FEEL IT

Working your entire body.

1. Place 2 cones about 4 yards apart. Starting at one cone with the other out to your side, stand in an athletic base position with a stretched bungee attached at your waist.
2. With resistance from the bungee, shuffle laterally away to the next cone, pushing with your outside leg and picking up with your inside foot.
3. Immediately reverse direction and repeat the movement.
4. Without pausing, continue to shuffle back and forth for the remainder of the set.
5. Reverse the direction of the resistance and repeat.

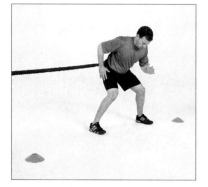
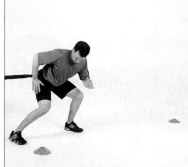
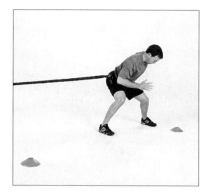

Lateral Shuffle—Resisted Quick and Stabilize

STEPS

1. Place 2 cones about 4 yards apart. Starting at one cone with the other out to your side, stand in an athletic base position with a stretched bungee attached at your waist.

2. With resistance from the bungee, shuffle laterally to the next cone, pushing with your outside leg and picking up with your inside foot.

3. Immediately reverse direction, shuffle back to the starting position, and pause for 3 seconds.

4. Complete the set on one side before reversing the direction of the resistance and repeating.

COACHING KEY
Do not allow your feet to come together. Minimize the amount of time during the change of direction.

FEEL IT
Working your entire body.

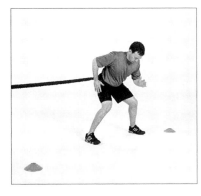
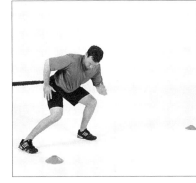
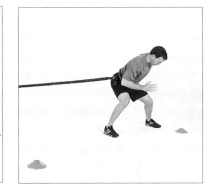

Sled March—Low

COACHING KEY
Extend your hips
with each step
and keep your
hips low and your
back flat.

FEEL IT
Working your
entire body.

STEPS

1. Stand in a split squat position with a sled attached to your waist.
2. March forward by pushing off the ground while leaning forward and keeping your hips as low as possible as your opposite arm swings forward.
3. Repeat the movement with your opposite arm and leg.
4. Continue alternating to complete the set.

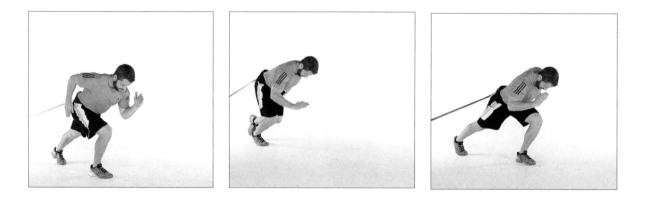

Chest Pass—1 Leg

STEPS

1. Stand in an athletic stance (quarter squat) on one leg 3 to 4 feet in front of a wall, holding a medicine ball at chest level with your arms straight.
2. Bring the ball to your chest and then immediately throw it as hard as possible against the wall.
3. Catch the ball and immediately go into your next throw.
4. Continue for the prescribed number of repetitions, switch legs and repeat to complete the set.

COACHING KEY
Keep your chest up, standing knee slightly bent, and hips back.

FEEL IT
Working your entire body.

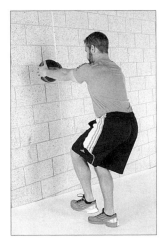
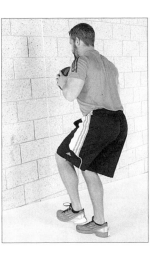
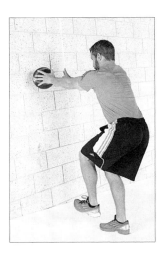
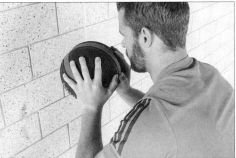

Chest Pass—Split Squat

COACHING KEY

Do not let your back knee touch the ground.

FEEL IT

Working your entire body.

STEPS

1. Stand in a low split stance 3 to 4 feet in front of a wall, holding a medicine ball at chest level with your arms straight.
2. Bring the ball to your chest and then immediately throw it as hard as possible against the wall.
3. Catch the ball and immediately go into your next throw.
4. Continue for the remainder of the set, switching legs halfway.

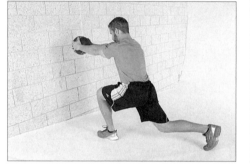
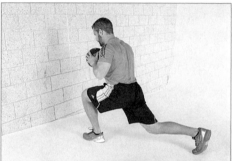
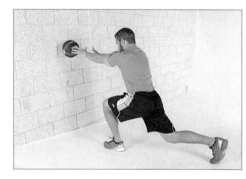
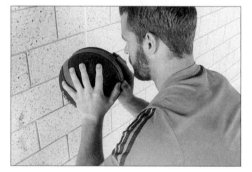

Chest Pass—Standing

STEPS

1. Stand in an athletic stance 3 to 4 feet in front of a wall, holding a medicine ball at chest level with your arms straight.
2. Bring the ball to your chest and then immediately throw it as hard as possible against the wall.
3. Catch the ball and immediately go into your next throw.
4. Continue for the remainder of the set.

COACHING KEY

Keep your chest up, knees slightly bent, and hips back.

FEEL IT

Working your entire body.

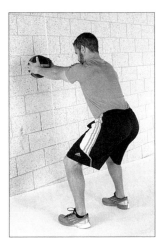
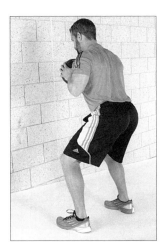
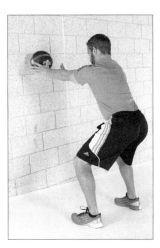

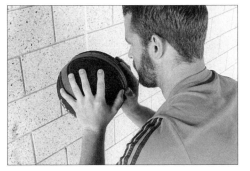

Granny Toss

COACHING KEY

Extend through your hips and arms while keeping your chest up.

FEEL IT

Working your entire body.

STEPS

1. Stand in an athletic stance with your knees slightly bent and hips back, holding a medicine ball above your head with straight arms.
2. Keeping your arms straight, lower yourself into a squat as you reach the ball down between your legs.
3. Explode out of the squat by jumping vertically and launching the medicine ball straight up as high as possible.
4. Let the ball bounce to a rest, pick it up, and return to the starting position.
5. Continue for the remainder of the set.

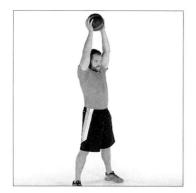 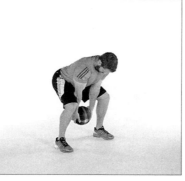 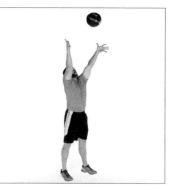

Overhead Pass—1 Leg

STEPS

1. Stand 1 to 2 feet away from a wall balancing on one leg with your feet shoulder-width apart, holding a medicine ball overhead.
2. Cock the ball behind your head and immediately throw it against the wall by driving your elbows down.
3. Catch the ball above your head and immediately repeat.
4. Continue for the prescribed number of repetitions, switch legs and repeat to complete the set.

COACHING KEY
Keep your chest up, stomach tight, and torso still.

FEEL IT
Working your torso, legs, and arms.

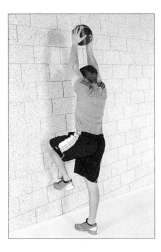
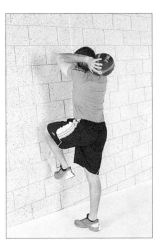
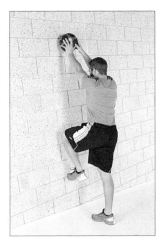

Overhead Pass—Split Squat

STEPS

1. Stand 1 to 2 feet away from a wall in a low split stance, with your feet shoulder-width apart, holding a medicine ball overhead.
2. Cock the ball behind your head and immediately throw it against the wall by driving your elbows down.
3. Catch the ball above your head and immediately repeat.
4. Continue for the prescribed number of repetitions, switch legs and repeat to complete the set.

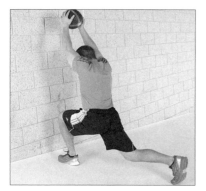 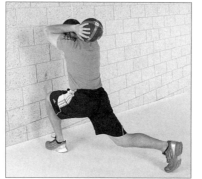 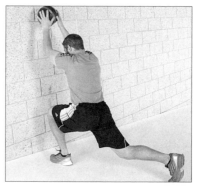

Overhead Throw

1. Stand perpendicular to a wall and about 10 yards away, holding a medicine ball with two hands at your waist.
2. Bend your knees and hips slightly as you bring the ball behind your back hip and rotate your shoulders away from the wall.
3. Drive off your back leg and step toward the wall as you bring the ball up the side of your body and throw it against the wall.
4. Collect the ball and return to the starting position.
5. Complete the set on one side before repeating on the other.

COACHING KEY
Throw the ball down as you throw it into the wall.

FEEL IT
Working your entire body.

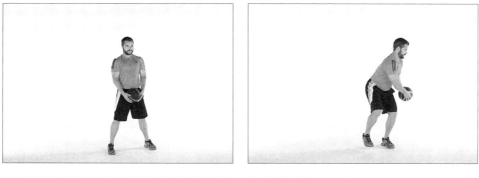

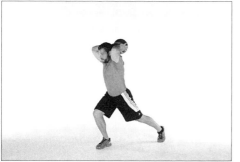

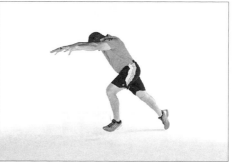

Parallel Rotational Throw—Kneeling

STEPS

1. Kneel on a soft mat or pad, facing a wall about 2 to 3 feet away, holding a medicine ball at waist level.

2. Rotate your shoulders, torso, and hips away from the wall, taking the ball behind your hip.

3. Throw the ball against the wall, initiating the move by rotating your hips, followed by your torso, arms, and the ball.

4. Catch the ball and immediately begin your next throw.

5. Complete the set on one side before repeating on the other.

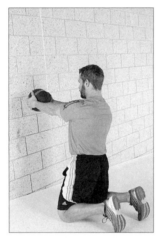 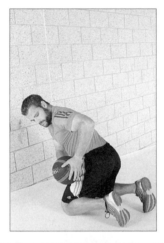 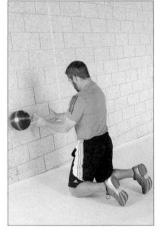

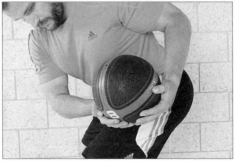

Parallel Rotational Throw—Split Squat

STEPS

1. Stand in a low split stance facing a wall about 2 to 3 feet away, holding a medicine ball at waist level.
2. Rotate your shoulders and torso over your front leg, taking the ball behind your hip.
3. Rotating your shoulders and torso back toward the wall, throw the ball at the wall.
4. Catch the ball and immediately throw back into the wall.
5. Complete the set on one side before switching legs and repeating on the other side.

COACHING KEY
Do not let your back knee touch the ground.

FEEL IT
Working your entire body.

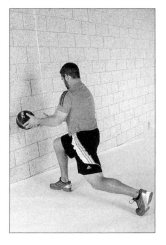
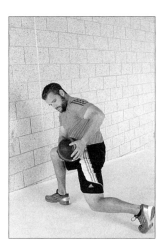
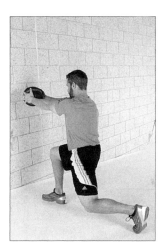

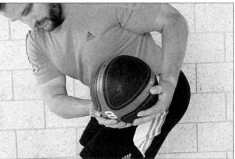

Parallel Rotational Throw—Standing

COACHING KEY
Initiate the throw
with your hips.

FEEL IT
Working your
entire body.

STEPS

1. Stand in an athletic stance with your feet slightly wider than shoulder-width apart, facing a wall about 2 to 3 feet away, holding a medicine ball at waist level.
2. Rotate your shoulders, torso, and hips away from the wall, taking the ball behind your hip.
3. Initiate the throw by exploding your hip back toward the wall and follow with your torso, arms, and the ball.
4. Catch the ball with your arms slightly bent and immediately go into your next repetition.
5. Complete the set on one side before repeating on the other side.

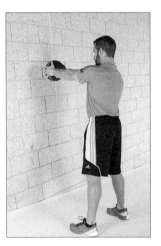
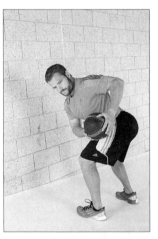
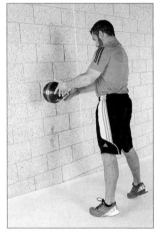
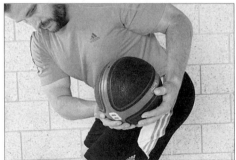

Perpendicular Rotational Throw—1 Leg

STEPS

1. Stand perpendicular to a wall about 2 to 3 feet away on your outside leg, holding a medicine ball in front of your body.
2. Rotate your torso away from the wall as you drop into a single-leg squat, taking the ball behind your back hip.
3. Rotating your shoulders and torso, throw the ball at the wall as your inside knee drives forward.
4. Catch the ball and immediately begin your next throw.
5. Complete the set on one side before switching legs and repeating on the other side.

COACHING KEY
Initiate the throw with your hips.

FEEL IT
Working your entire body.

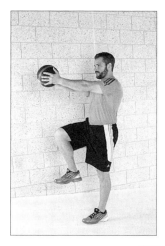
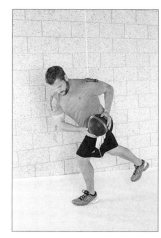
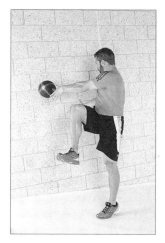
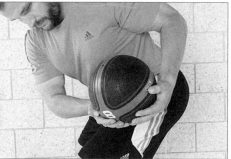

Perpendicular Rotational Throw— Standing

STEPS

1. Stand in an athletic stance with your feet slightly wider than shoulder-width apart, your side to a wall about 2 to 3 feet away, holding a medicine ball at waist level.
2. Rotate your torso and hips away from the wall, taking the ball behind your back hip.
3. Throw the ball against the wall, initiating the move by rotating your hips, followed by your torso, arms, and the ball.
4. Catch the ball and immediately begin your next throw.
5. Complete the set on one side before repeating on the other side.

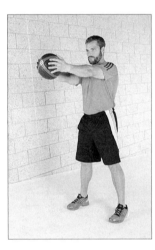 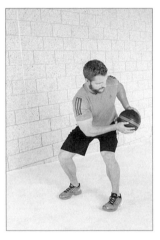 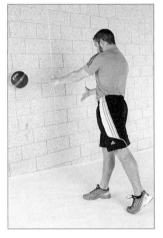

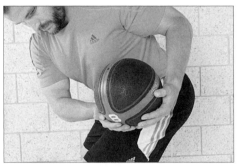

Walking Lunge to Chest Pass

STEPS

1. Stand holding a medicine ball in front of your chest with your arms bent.
2. Step forward into a lunge and immediately explode out, lunging up and forward as you press and release the medicine ball as far as you can into the air at a 45-degree angle.
3. Let the ball bounce to a rest.
4. Retrieve the ball, return to the starting position, and repeat the movement with the opposite foot forward.
5. Continue alternating to complete the set.

COACHING KEY
Drive off your front leg as you lunge forward.

FEEL IT
Working your entire body.

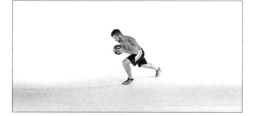
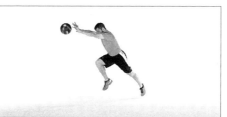

Walking Lunge to Chest Pass—Non-Countermovement

1. Stand in a low split stance holding a medicine ball in front of your chest with your arms bent.
2. Explode out, lunging up and forward as you press and release the medicine ball as far as you can into the air at a 45-degree angle.
3. Let the ball bounce to a rest.
4. Retrieve the ball, return to the starting position, and repeat the movement with the opposite foot forward.
5. Continue alternating to complete the set.

COACHING KEY

Drive off your front leg as you lunge forward.

FEEL IT

Working your entire body.

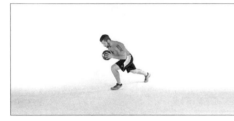
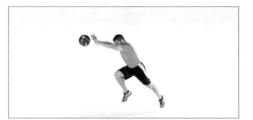

Cable Chop—
Lateral, Half Kneeling

STEPS

1. Attach a rope handle to the high pulley of a cable machine and grab it with both hands. Begin in a half-kneeling position with your side to the machine, your outside knee down, and your inside foot on the floor.
2. In one fluid motion, turn your hips and shoulders away from the machine, pull the handle to your chest, then push the rope down and away from you.
3. Reverse the pattern to the starting position.
4. Complete the set on one side before repeating with the other side.

COACHING KEY
Keep your chest up and turn toward and away from the machine with each repetition.

FEEL IT
Working your hips, shoulders, triceps, and abdominals.

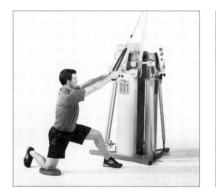
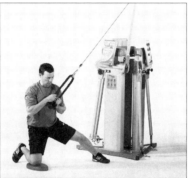
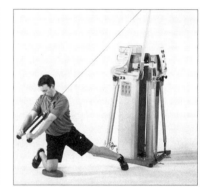

Hang Snatch

COACHING KEY

As you pull the weight upward, you should feel as if you're jumping, so that your ankles, knees, and hips fully extend. Do not begin to pull with the upper body until the hips are fully extended.

FEEL IT

Working your entire body.

STEPS

1. Stand holding a barbell straight down in front of your body with your feet shoulder-width apart.
2. Keeping your back flat and chest up, push your hips back and down to lower the weight just above your knees.
3. In one explosive motion, extend your hips as quickly as possible, pulling the weight straight up.
4. Allow the barbell to float upward. When the weight reaches its maximum height, drop your body underneath and "catch" it overhead.
5. Lower the weight back to the starting position.
6. Continue to complete the set.

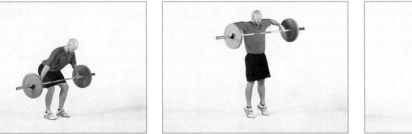
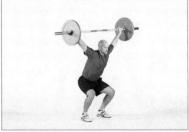

Hang Snatch Pull

STEPS

1. Stand with your feet shoulder-width apart in front of a barbell with a wide overhand grip (palms facing toward you).
2. Keeping your back flat and chest up, push your hips back and down to lower the weight below your knees.
3. In one explosive motion, extend your hips as quickly as possible.
4. Lower the weight back to the starting position.
5. Continue to complete the set.

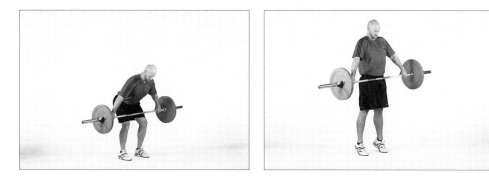

COACHING KEY

As you pull the weight upward, you should feel as if you're jumping, so that your ankles, knees, and hips fully extend. Do not begin to pull with the upper body until the hips are fully extended.

FEEL IT

Working your entire body.

Hang Snatch—1 Arm (Dumbbell)

COACHING KEY

As you pull the weight upward, you should feel as if you're jumping, so that your ankles, knees, and hips fully extend.

FEEL IT

Working your entire body.

STEPS

1. Stand holding a dumbbell straight down in front of your body, with your feet shoulder-width apart.
2. Keeping your back flat and chest up, push your hips back and dip down at the knees to lower the weight below your knees.
3. In one explosive motion, extend your hips as quickly as possible, pulling the weight straight up.
4. Allow the dumbbell to float upward. When the weight reaches its maximum height, drop your body underneath and "catch" it overhead.
5. Lower the weight back to the starting position.
6. Complete the set on one side before repeating with the opposite arm.

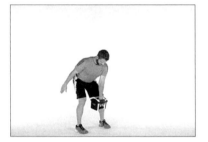 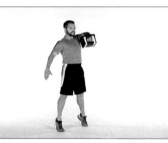 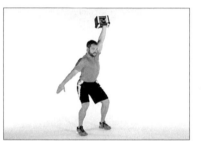

Kettlebell Swing

STEPS

1. Stand holding a kettlebell with both hands in front of you with straight arms.
2. Drop your hips back and down into a squat as you lower the kettlebell along an arc under and between your legs.
3. Initiating the movement with your hips, explosively drive your hips and swing the kettlebell up until your arms are parallel to the floor.
4. Without pausing, continue for the full set.

COACHING KEY

Keep your arms straight and your shoulder blades back and down throughout the movement.

FEEL IT

Working your glutes, hamstrings, and back.

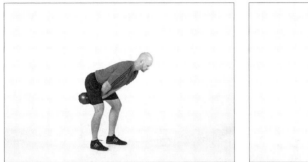

Overhead Rotational Squat—1 Arm (Kettlebell)

STEPS

1. Stand holding a kettlebell in one hand pressed straight above the same-side shoulder.
2. Initiating the move with your hips, squat back and down as you rotate your shoulders to the same side as the kettlebell and reach straight down to touch your foot with the other hand.
3. Reverse the movement pattern to return to the starting position.
4. Complete the set on one side before repeating on the opposite side.

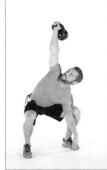

COACHING KEY

Keep your back flat and chest up throughout the movement.

FEEL IT

Working your entire body.

Overhead Slam (Medicine Ball)

STEPS

1. Stand in an athletic stance with your knees slightly bent and hips back, holding a medicine ball at waist level.
2. Extend your hips and stand tall as you bring the ball above and behind your head.
3. Explode down and throw the ball into the ground.
4. Let the ball bounce, pick it up, and return to the starting position.
5. Continue for the remainder of the set.

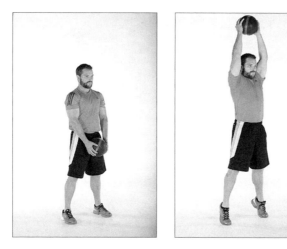
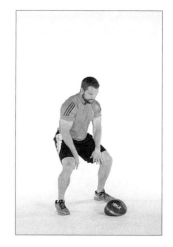

Overhead Squat (Slide)

1. Stand tall with your feet on slides and a miniband looped around your wrists with your arms straight overhead and pulled apart to create tension in the band.
2. Maintaining tension on the miniband and initiating the move with your hips, squat back and down until your thighs are close to parallel to the floor or the slides are about to begin to move.
3. Return to a standing position by pushing through your hips.
4. Continue for prescribed number of repetitions.

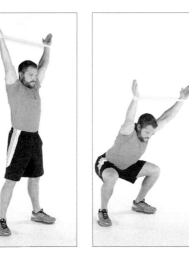

COACHING KEY
Keep your back flat, tension on the miniband, and do not let the slides move as you squat down.

FEEL IT
Working your entire body.

Push Press

COACHING KEY

Initiate the movement with your legs; do not push the weights with your arms until your hips are fully extended.

FEEL IT

Working your entire body.

STEPS

1. Stand holding a barbell on the front of your shoulders.
2. Dip down at the hips and knees.
3. Immediately explode back up, pressing the bar overhead by extending your hips without letting your knees collapse to the inside.
4. "Catch" the bar overhead with your arms straight and hips and knees extended.
5. Slowly lower the weights back to the starting position.
6. Continue for the remainder of the set.

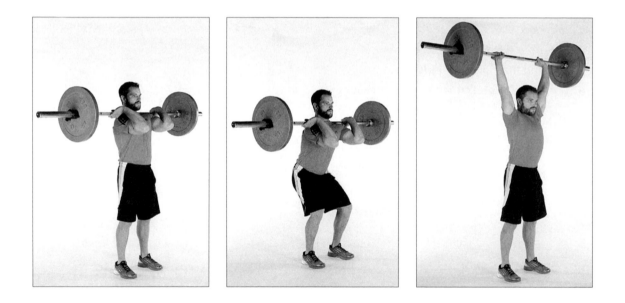

Reverse Lunge to Row (Cable)

1. Stand facing a cable machine holding a handle attached to midpulley position in one hand.
2. Step back into a lunge with the same-side leg as the cable handle as you reach the arm holding the cable forward.
3. Push through your hip to return to a standing position as you pull the cable handle to your body.
4. Complete the set on one side before repeating on the opposite arm and leg.

COACHING KEY

Keep your back flat and drive through your glutes as you return to a standing position.

FEEL IT

Working the glutes and hamstrings of the front leg and the shoulder of the arm holding the handle.

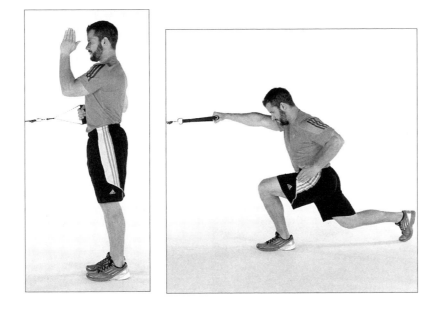

Romanian Deadlift [RDL] to Row— 1 Arm, 1 Leg (Cable)

STEPS

1. Stand on one leg facing a cable machine while holding a handle attached to midpulley position in the same-side hand at your side.

2. Keeping your standing knee slightly bent, hinge at the hip while reaching your handle hand forward and the opposite leg straight behind you.

3. Contract your glutes and hamstrings to return to a standing position as you pull the handle to your body.

4. Complete the set on one side before repeating on the opposite arm and leg.

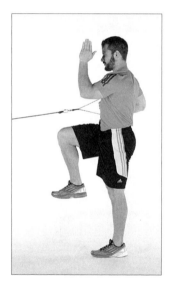
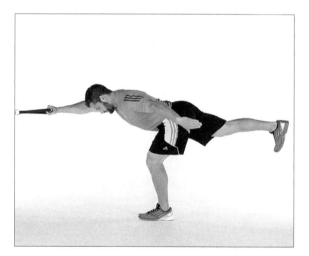

Rotational Chop—1 Arm, Standing, Reactive

STEPS

1. Attach a rope handle to the high pulley of a cable machine and grab it with your outside hand. Stand with your side to the machine and your outside arm across your body toward the pulley.
2. In one fluid motion, push off your inside foot, turn your hips and shoulders away from the machine, pull the handle to your chest, then push the rope down and away from you.
3. Immediately reverse the pattern back to the starting position.
4. As quickly as possible, continue for the remainder of the set.
5. Repeat the set on the opposite side and arm.

COACHING KEY

Keep your chest up, turning toward and away from the machine with each repetition.

FEEL IT

Working your hips, shoulders, triceps, and abdominals.

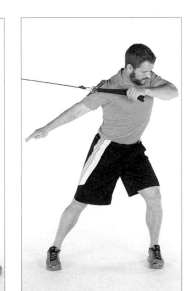
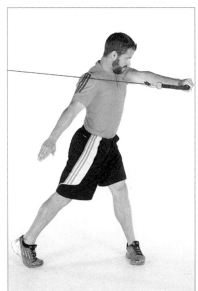

Rotational Chop—Standing

STEPS

1. Attach a rope handle to the high pulley of a cable machine and grab it with both hands. Stand with your side to the machine and your arms across your body toward the handle.
2. In one fluid motion, push off your inside foot, turn your hips and shoulders away from the machine, pull the handle to your chest, then push the rope down and away from you.
3. Reverse the pattern to the starting position.
4. Continue for the remainder of the set before repeating with the opposite side.

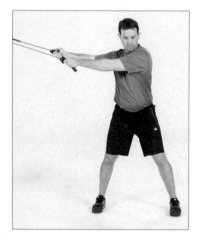
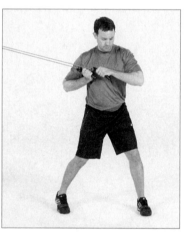
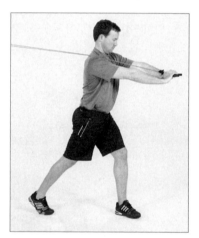

Rotational Lift

STEPS

1. Attach a rope to the low pulley of a cable machine. Stand with your side to the cable machine, holding the rope with both hands, feet slightly wider than shoulder-width apart.
2. Rotate your hips and shoulders toward the machine as you lower your hips toward the ground.
3. In one continuous motion, explode out of this position as you press through your inside leg, pull the handles toward your chest, rotate away from the machine, and push the rope up and away from the machine.
4. Reverse the movement pattern back to the starting position.
5. Continue for the remainder of the set before repeating on the opposite side.

COACHING KEY

Turn toward and away from the machine with each repetition. Keep your inside elbow up, making sure the cable travels underneath your arm.

FEEL IT

Working your shoulders, triceps, torso, and hips.

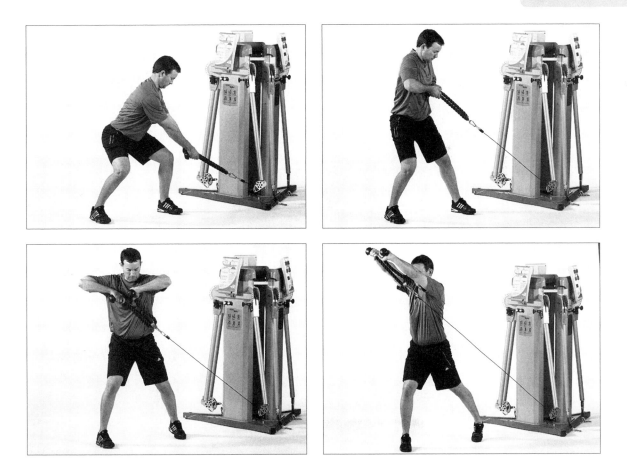

Rotational Lift—Reactive

1. Attach a rope to the low pulley of a cable machine. Stand with your side to the cable machine, holding the rope with both hands, feet slightly wider than shoulder-width apart.
2. Rotate your hips and shoulders toward the machine as you lower your hips toward the ground.
3. In one continuous motion, explode out of this position as you press through your inside leg, pull the handles toward your chest, rotate away from the machine, and push the rope up and away from the machine.
4. Immediately reverse the movement pattern back to the starting position.
5. As quickly as possible, continue for the remainder of the set.
6. Repeat the set on the opposite side.

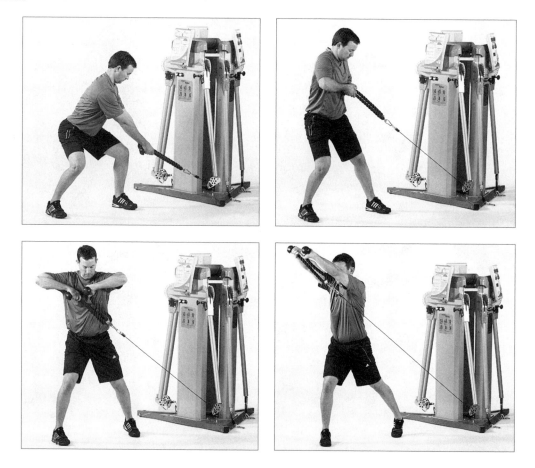

Rotational Push/Pull

1. Attach a handle to each side of two chest-high pulleys on a cable machine. Stand between the cable arms with your side to the machine, feet slightly wider than shoulder-width apart.
2. Hold the front handle with your outstretched outside arm and the back handle at your chest with your inside arm.
3. Sit your hips back and down into a half-squat position.
4. In one continuous motion, explode out of this position as you push your inside hip forward, press your inside hand away from your chest, and pull your outside hand toward your chest.
5. Reverse the movement pattern back to the starting position.
6. Complete the set on one side before repeating on the other side.

COACHING KEY
Keep your torso stable and avoid excessive shoulder rotation.

FEEL IT
Working your shoulders, triceps, torso, and hips.

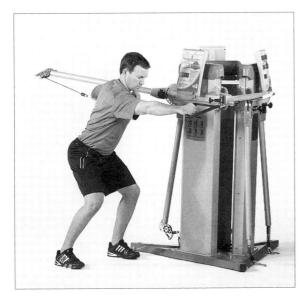 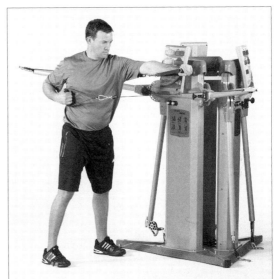

Rotational Push/Pull—Reactive

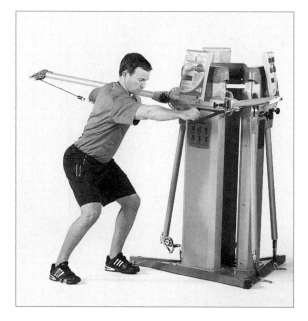

COACHING KEY
Keep your torso stable and avoid excessive shoulder rotation.

FEEL IT
Working your shoulders, triceps, torso, and hips.

STEPS

1. Attach a handle to each side of two chest-high pulleys on a cable machine. Stand between the cable arms with your side to the machine, feet slightly wider than shoulder-width apart.
2. Hold the front handle with an outstretched outside arm and the back handle at your chest with your inside arm.
3. Sit your hips back and down into a half-squat position.
4. In one continuous motion, explode out of this position as you push your inside hip forward, press your inside hand away from your chest, and pull your outside hand toward your chest.
5. Immediately reverse the movement pattern back to the starting position.
6. As quickly as possible, continue for the remainder of the set.
7. Repeat the set on the opposite side.

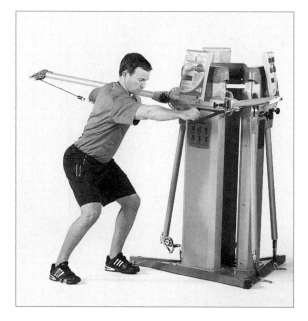
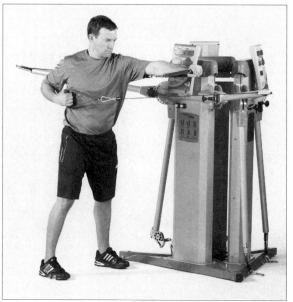

Rotational Row

1. Attach a handle to the low pulley of a cable machine. Stand with your side to the machine, holding the cable at your side with your outside hand, feet slightly wider than shoulder-width apart.
2. Rotate your hips and shoulders toward the machine as you sit back and down, reaching the handle across your body toward the pulley.
3. In one smooth motion, rotate your outside shoulder back, pull the handle to your outside hip, and push up and away from the machine with your inside leg.
4. Reverse the movement back to the starting position.
5. Complete the set on one side before repeating on the other side.

COACHING KEY

Turn your hips and shoulders toward and away from the machine with each repetition.

FEEL IT

Working your arms, shoulders, upper back, torso, and legs.

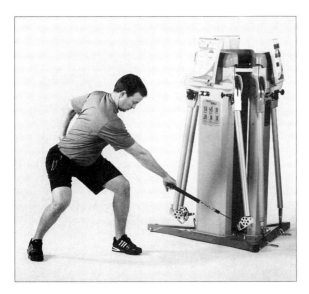
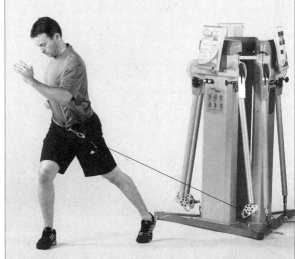

STEPS

1. Attach a handle to the low pulley of a cable machine. Stand with your side to the machine, holding the cable at your side with your outside hand, feet slightly wider than shoulder-width apart.

2. Rotate your hips and shoulders toward the machine as you sit back and down, reaching the handle across your body toward the pulley.

3. In one smooth motion, rotate your outside shoulder back, pull the handle to your outside hip, and push up and away from the machine with your inside leg.

4. Immediately reverse the pattern back to the starting position.

5. As quickly as possible, continue for the remainder of the set.

6. Repeat the set on the opposite side and arm.

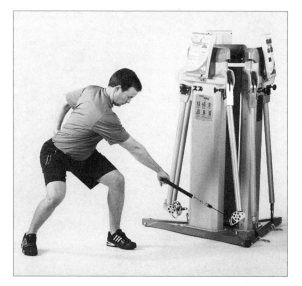
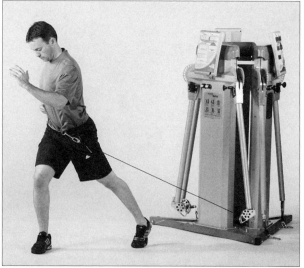

Shoulder Press with Lateral Flexion (Kettlebell)

STEPS

1. Stand with your feet wider than shoulder-width apart, holding a kettlebell in one hand at your shoulder.
2. Side-bend your torso toward the kettlebell side and extend your opposite arm straight up.
3. Side-bend your torso away from the kettlebell side and lift the kettlebell straight up as you reach straight down to your foot with the other hand.
4. Reverse the movement pattern back to the starting position
5. Complete the set on one side before repeating with the kettlebell in the opposite hand.

COACHING KEY

Keep your chest up, back flat, and legs straight throughout the movement.

FEEL IT

Working your shoulders and torso.

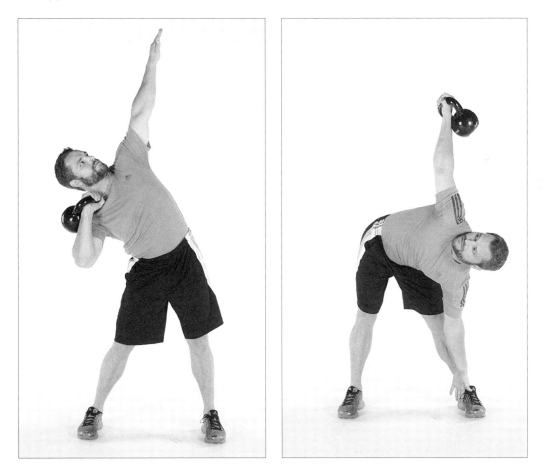

Squat to Press Throw

COACHING KEY

Generate power from your lower body; don't just rely on your upper body to throw the ball.

FEEL IT

Working your entire body.

STEPS

1. Stand in an athletic position with your feet shoulder-width apart, holding a medicine ball at chest level.
2. Squat by sitting your hips back and down, keeping your weight in the middle of your arches.
3. Extend powerfully through your hips, vertically launching the ball and your body into the air.
4. Let the ball bounce to a rest.
5. Pick up the ball and return to the starting position.
6. Continue for the remainder of the set.

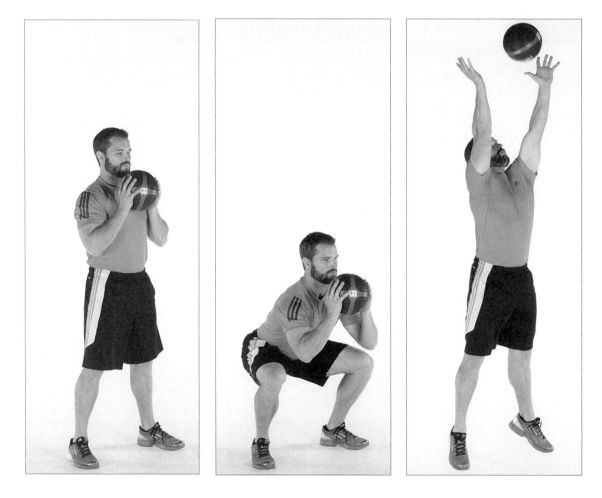

Squat to Press—1 Arm (Dumbbell)

1. Stand with your feet shoulder-width apart, holding a dumbbell at one shoulder with your elbow pointed down.
2. Initiating the movement with your hips, squat back and down until your thighs are parallel to the floor.
3. Stand by pushing through your hips and press the dumbbell overhead.
4. Lower the weight and return to the starting position.
5. Complete the set with one arm before repeating with the opposite arm.

COACHING KEY
Keep your shoulders parallel to the floor and maintain your posture as you press the dumbbell overhead.

FEEL IT
Working your glutes, hamstrings, quads, and shoulders.

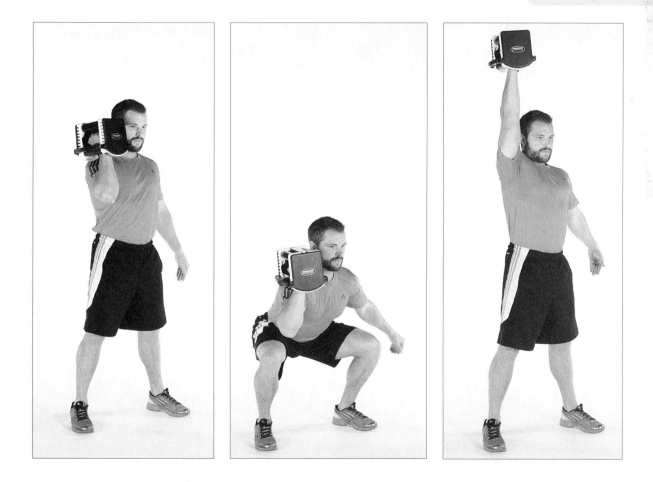

Stability Chop—Half Kneeling (Cable)

STEPS

1. Attach a bar to the high pulley of a cable machine and grab it with both hands. With your side to the machine, get in a half-kneeling position, with your inside foot up and outside knee on a soft mat or pad.
2. With your outside hand low and inside hand high on the bar, let your arms go in toward the machine.
3. Pull the bar diagonally down and across your body and continue by pressing your inside arm down as you draw your outside arm behind you.
4. Reverse the movement back to the starting position.
5. Complete the set on one side before repeating on the other side.

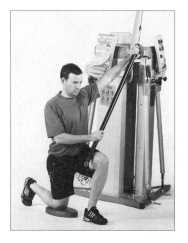
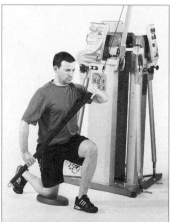
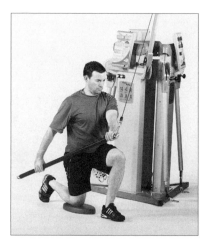

Stability Lift—Half Kneeling (Cable)

1. Attach a bar to the low pulley of a cable machine and grab it with both hands. With your side to the machine, get in a half-kneeling position, with your outside foot up and inside knee on a soft mat or pad.
2. With your inside hand low and outside hand high on the bar, let your arms go in toward the machine.
3. Pull the bar diagonally up and across your body, and then press it straight up with your inside arm above your inside shoulder.
4. Reverse the movement back to the starting position.
5. Complete the set on one side before repeating on the other side.

COACHING KEY
Do not allow any movement in your torso during the exercise.

FEEL IT
Working your shoulders and torso.

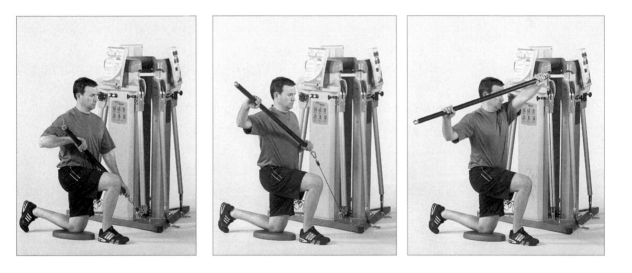

Turkish Get-Up (Kettlebell)

COACHING KEY
Keep your back
flat throughout the
movement.

FEEL IT
Working your
entire body.

STEPS

1. Start in a fetal position holding a kettlebell in front of your chest with your bottom hand, top hand resting on the handle.

2. Roll onto your back so that you are holding the kettlebell in one hand resting on your shoulder and the opposite arm at your side at 45 degrees. Keep the same-side leg of the kettlebell bent with your foot flat on the ground.

3. Press the kettlebell straight up into the air above your shoulder.

4. Keeping the foot of the bent leg flat on the floor, sit up, supporting your upper body with your opposite arm in a straight position.

5. With the kettlebell still pressed above your shoulder, push your hips off the ground and pull your straight leg underneath your body into a kneeling position.

6. With the kettlebell still pressed above your shoulder, bring the kettlebell-side foot forward into a half-kneeling position.

7. With the kettlebell still pressed above your shoulder, push through your hips and stand up.

8. Reverse the movement pattern to return to the starting position.

9. Complete the set on one side before repeating on the opposite side.

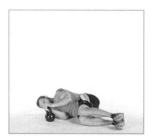
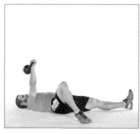
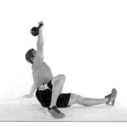
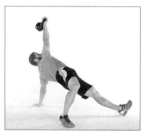

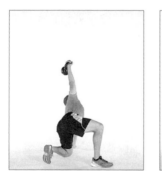
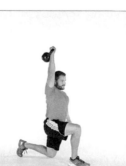
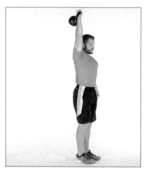

Bench Press (Barbell)

`STEPS`

1. Lie faceup on a bench holding a barbell straight over your chest with an overhand grip (palms facing forward).
2. Lower the bar to your chest under control.
3. Press the weight back up to the starting position.
4. Continue for the full set.

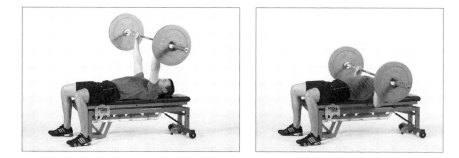

Bench Press (Dumbbell)

`STEPS`

1. Lie faceup on a bench holding dumbbells at your shoulders with an overhand grip (palms facing forward).
2. Press the weights straight up over your chest.
3. Lower the dumbbells until your upper arms just break parallel to the ground.
4. Continue for the remainder of the set.

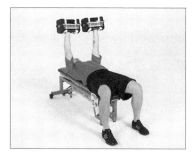
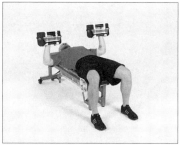

Bench Press—1 Arm (Dumbbell)

Keep your
stomach tight
and don't let
anything move
except your arm.

FEEL IT

Working your
chest and torso.

STEPS

1. Lie with your right glute and shoulder blade on a bench and your left glute and shoulder blade off.

2. Hold a dumbbell straight above you in your left hand while reaching your right hand to the ceiling.

3. Lower the dumbbell until your upper arm is parallel with the ground.

4. Press the weight back to the starting position.

5. Complete the set on one side before repeating with the opposite arm.

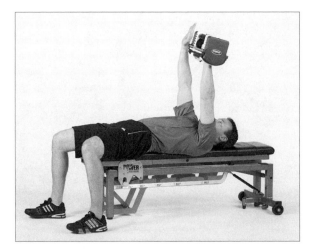

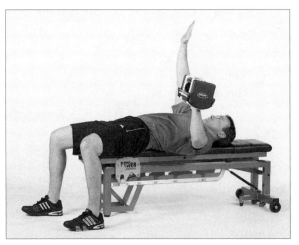

Bench Press—1 Arm, Off Bench

1. Lie faceup on a bench holding a dumbbell at your shoulder in one hand, with the other hand reaching straight to the ceiling. Only your shoulders should be on the bench and your hips should be parallel to the ground.
2. Keeping your hips bridged up, press the dumbbell over your chest.
3. Lower the weight back to your shoulder until your upper arm is parallel to the floor.
4. Complete the set on one side before repeating with the opposite arm.

COACHING KEY
Contract your glutes and keep your stomach tight to stabilize your torso.

FEEL IT
Working your glutes, torso, chest, shoulders, and triceps.

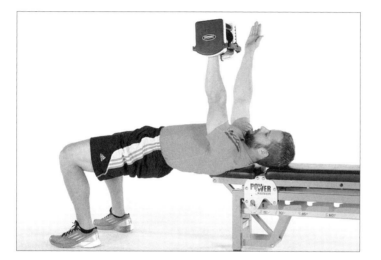

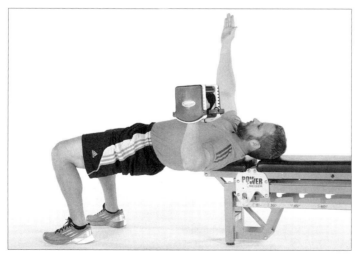

Bench Press—Alternating Dumbbell with Leg Lowering

COACHING KEY

Keep your stomach tight and your hips and shoulders on the bench at all times.

FEEL IT

Working your chest, shoulder, and triceps.

STEPS

1. Lie faceup on a bench holding dumbbells straight over your chest with an overhand grip (palms facing forward) and your hips and knees flexed to 90 degrees. This exercise can also be done wearing ankle weights.

2. Lower a dumbbell in one hand until your upper arm just breaks parallel to the ground as you lower your opposite leg toward the ground, keeping your knee bent to 90 degrees.

3. Press the weight up and lift your leg back to the starting position.

4. Repeat the movement with your opposite arm and leg.

5. Continue alternating to complete the set.

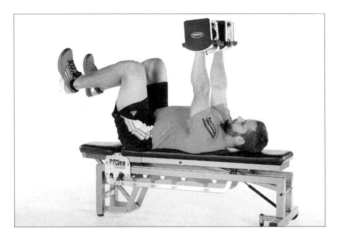

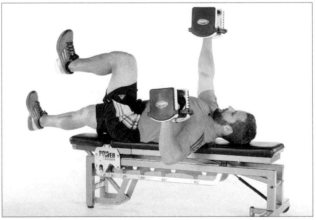

Incline Bench Press—Alternating (Dumbbell)

STEPS

1. Lie faceup on an incline bench holding dumbbells straight over your chest with an overhand grip (palms facing forward).
2. Keeping your right arm straight, lower the dumbbell in your left hand until your upper arm just breaks parallel to the ground.
3. Return to the starting position and repeat on the other side.
4. Continue alternating to complete the set.

COACHING KEY

Keep your feet on the floor, your stomach tight, and your hips and shoulders on the bench at all times.

FEEL IT

Working your chest, shoulder, and triceps.

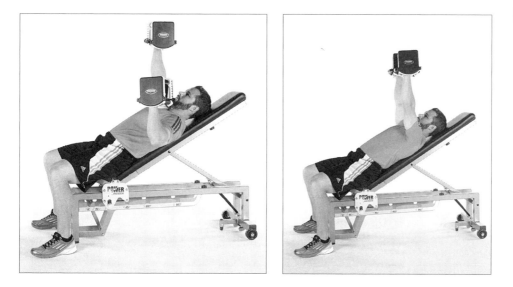

Push-Up

1. Start in the classic push-up position, with your hands beneath your shoulders and your legs straight behind you.
2. Keeping your torso stable and hips square to the ground, bend your elbows to lower your body toward the ground.
3. Without touching the ground with your torso or knees, push yourself back up.
4. Continue for the full set.

COACHING KEY

Keep your body in a straight line and push your chest as far away from your hands as possible.

FEEL IT

Working your chest, arms, and torso.

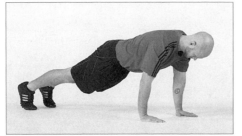 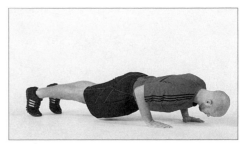

Push-Up (TRX)

STEPS

1. Start in a push-up position, with your hands directly beneath your shoulders and inside a TRX strap so that the TRX hangs vertically. Place your feet shoulder-width apart and lean your body forward.
2. Keeping your torso stable and hips square to the ground, bend your elbows to lower your torso toward the ground.
3. When your elbows are bent to about 90 degrees, push yourself back up.
4. Continue for the full set.

COACHING KEY

Pull your toes toward your shins and maintain a straight line from ears to ankles.

FEEL IT

Working your chest, arms, and torso.

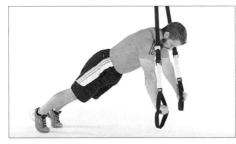 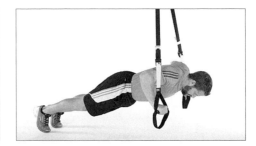

Push-Up on Bench—Countermovement (Plyometric)

STEPS

1. Start in a modified push-up position, with your hands on a bench.
2. Lower your chest to the bench.
3. Immediately drive up your body explosively so that your arms are fully extended and your hands are off the bench as far as possible.
4. Upon landing, reset to the starting position.
5. Continue for the remainder of the set.

COACHING KEY

Keep your body in a straight line throughout the movement.

FEEL IT

Working your chest, shoulders, and arms.

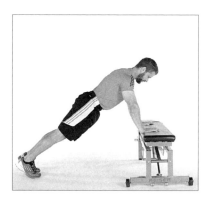
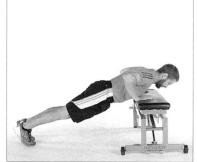
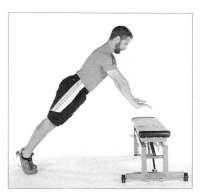

Bent-Over Row—1 Arm (Dumbbell)

STEPS

1. Stand hinged over at the waist holding a dumbbell in one hand. Hold on to a waist-high object with your other hand for support.
2. Slide your shoulder blade back and then drive your elbow toward the ceiling, pulling the weight up toward the side of your rib cage.
3. Lower the weight back to the starting position.
4. Complete the set on one side before repeating with the opposite arm.

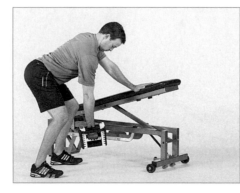 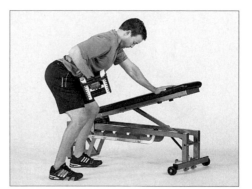

Bent-Over Row—1 Arm, 1 Leg (Dumbbell—Contralateral)

STEPS

1. Stand on one leg holding a dumbbell in your opposite hand. Hold on to a waist-high object with your other hand for balance.
2. Hinge forward at the waist while extending your leg back behind you until it's parallel to the floor.
3. Slide your shoulder blade back and then drive your elbow toward the ceiling, pulling the weight up toward the side of your rib cage.
4. Lower the weight back to the starting position.
5. Complete the set on one side before repeating on the opposite leg and arm.

COACHING KEY

Keep your back, shoulders, and non-standing leg parallel to the floor.

FEEL IT

Working your upper back, lats, and shoulders.

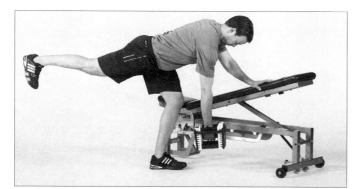

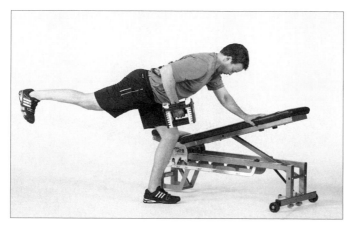

Bent-Over Row—1 Arm, 1 Leg (Dumbbell—Ipsilateral)

STEPS

1. Stand on one leg holding a dumbbell in the hand of the same side. Place your free hand on a waist-high object for balance.
2. Hinge forward at the waist while extending your leg back behind you until it's parallel to the floor.
3. Slide your shoulder blade back and then drive your elbow toward the ceiling, pulling the weight up toward the side of your rib cage.
4. Lower the weight back to the starting position.
5. Complete the set on one side before repeating with the opposite leg and arm.

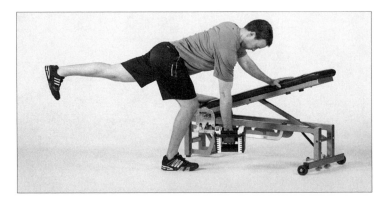

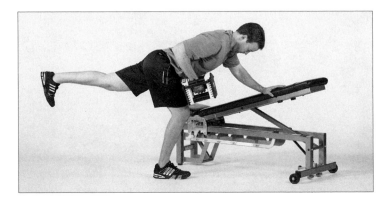

Pulldown—Alternating

1. Sit under a lat pulldown machine, holding a pair of handles overhead with your palms facing away.
2. Keeping your torso stable, your chest up, and your shoulder blades back and down, pull your arms down so that the handles are at shoulder level.
3. Allow one arm to slowly straighten overhead.
4. Pull the handle back to shoulder level.
5. Repeat the movement with your opposite arm.
6. Continue alternating to complete the set.

COACHING KEY

Initiate the movement by sliding your shoulder blades back and down, and then drive your elbows toward the floor.

FEEL IT

Working your back and arms.

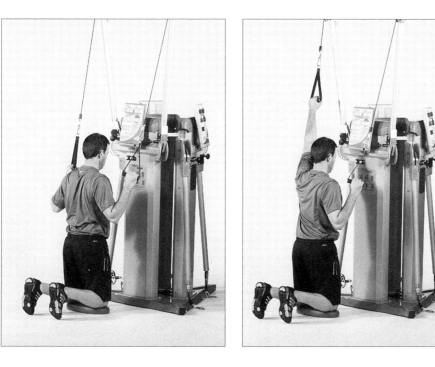

Pullover Extension—Alternating Dumbbell with Hip Extension

COACHING KEY

Lower the weight in a two-part motion—first from the elbow and then from the shoulder—and pull back to the start position in one fluid motion.

FEEL IT

Working your arms and torso.

STEPS

1. Lie faceup on a bench holding dumbbells in each hand with your arms straight over your shoulders and your hips and knees bent to 90 degrees.

2. Extend the hip and knee of one leg until your leg is straight while you lower the opposite-side dumbbell by bending your elbow to 90 degrees and then moving from your shoulder to continue lowering.

3. In one fluid motion, lift your leg back up while you drive your elbow back up and then straighten your arm to return to the starting position.

4. Repeat the movement with your opposite arm and leg.

5. Continue alternating to complete the set.

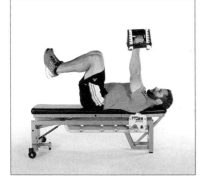 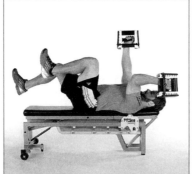 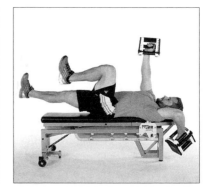

Pull-Up

1. Hang from a pull-up bar with either a neutral grip (palms facing each other) or overhand grip (palms facing out).
2. Keeping your legs still and initiating with your shoulder blades, pull your chest to the bar.
3. Lower yourself to the starting position.
4. Continue for the remainder of the set.

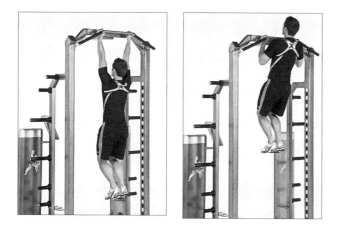

COACHING KEY
Straighten your arms completely at the end of the rep; at the top, think about driving your elbows back and down.

FEEL IT
Working your back and arms.

Pull-Up—3-Point Isometric Holds

1. Hang from a pull-up bar with either a neutral grip (palms facing each other) or overhand grip (palms facing out).
2. Keeping your legs still and initiating with your shoulder blades, pull your chest to the bar.
3. Lower your body a quarter of the way down and hold for the prescribed seconds.
4. Lower yourself down halfway and hold for the prescribed seconds again.
5. Lower yourself three-quarters of the way down and hold for the prescribed seconds.

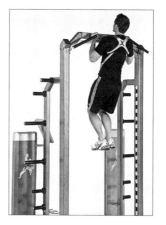

COACHING KEY
For added difficulty, wear a weight vest to add resistance.

FEEL IT
Working your back, shoulders, and arms.

Rotational Row (TRX)

STEPS

1. Secure two TRX straps together by looping one handle through the other. Hold them straight in front of your chest with one arm.
2. Keeping your legs straight and torso stable, lean backward so that the TRX straps hang diagonally.
3. Rotate the shoulder of the opposite arm away from the TRX straps.
4. In one continuous motion, rotate your shoulder forward and pull your chest toward the TRX straps.
5. Reverse the movement pattern to return to the starting position.
6. Complete the set on one side before repeating on the opposite arm.

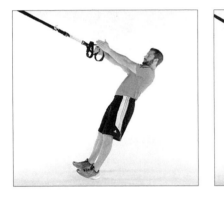
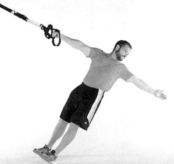
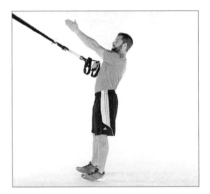

Front Squat (Barbell)

STEPS

1. Stand holding a barbell across the front of your shoulders with your palms facing you and your elbows up and in front of you.
2. Initiating the movement with your hips, squat back and down until your thighs are as close to parallel to the floor as possible.
3. Push through your hips and return to a standing position.
4. Continue for the full set.

COACHING KEY
Keep your chest up, back flat, and do not let your knees collapse to the inside.

FEEL IT
Working your glutes, hamstrings, and quads.

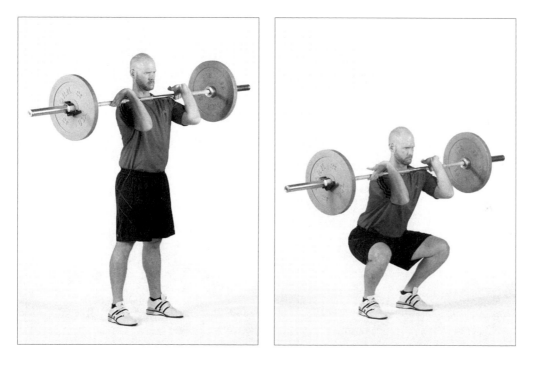

Lateral Lunge—Alternating (Dumbbell)

COACHING KEY

Keep your chest up and your back flat.

FEEL IT

Working your glutes, hamstrings, and quads and stretching the inner thigh of the straight leg.

STEPS

1. Stand holding a dumbbell in each hand by your sides.
2. Step to one side and lower your hips to the floor by squatting back and down with the stepping leg, keeping the other leg straight. The arms should remain still with one dumbbell on the outside of the squatting leg and one dumbbell between your legs.
3. Return to the starting position by pushing up with your bent leg.
4. Switch directions and repeat the movement.
5. Continue alternating to complete the set.

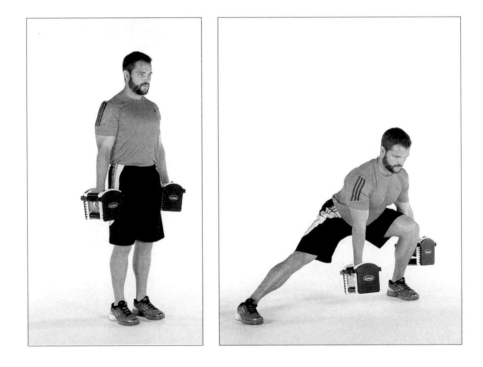

Lateral Lunge—Contralateral Bottom-Up Kettlebell (Slide)

STEPS

1. Stand with one foot on the ground and the other on a slide (or on a towel on a slippery surface) while holding a kettlebell by your head with the handle pointed down in the same-side hand as the foot on the slide.
2. Keeping your weight mostly on your foot on the ground, squat back and down through your hip and slide your opposite foot to the side, straightening your leg.
3. Stand up by pushing down with the standing leg.
4. Complete the set on one side before repeating with the opposite leg.

COACHING KEY

Think of this as a single-leg squat, placing the primary emphasis on the ground leg.

FEEL IT

Working the glute and quadriceps of the leg on the ground and stretching the groin of your sliding leg.

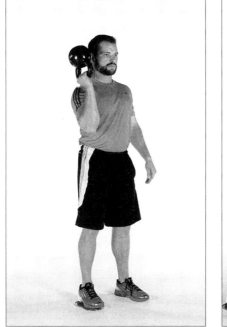
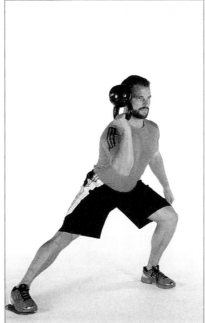

Lateral Lunge—Horizontal Resistance (Slide)

STEPS

1. Stand with one foot on the ground and the other on a slide (or on a towel on a slippery surface) and attached with an ankle strap to the low pulley on a cable machine.
2. Keeping your weight mostly on your foot on the ground, squat back and down through your hip and slide your opposite foot to the side, straightening your leg.
3. Stand up by pushing down with the standing leg.
4. Complete the set on one side before repeating with the opposite leg.

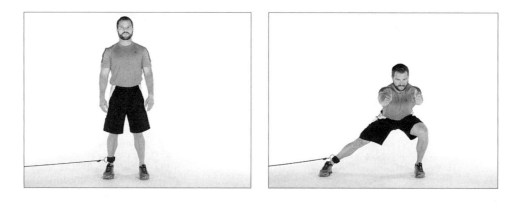

Reverse Lunge (Dumbbell)

STEPS

1. Stand tall with your feet about hip-width apart, holding a pair of dumbbells.
2. Keeping your chest up and your weight primarily on your front foot, step back into a lunge.
3. When your knee is just off the ground, push through your front hip to return to a standing position.
4. Repeat with the opposite leg.
5. Continue alternating to complete the set.

COACHING TIP
Do not let your front knee collapse to the inside, and don't let your back knee touch the ground.

FEEL IT
Working your glutes, hamstrings, and quads.

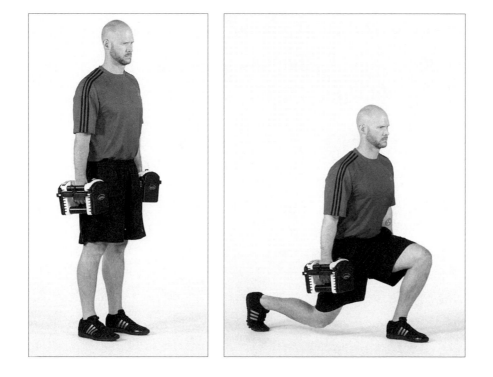

Reverse Lunge—Horizontal Resistance (Slide)

STEPS

1. Stand tall with your back to a cable machine with one foot flat on the floor, the other on a slide (or on a towel on a slippery surface), and a low-level cable attached to the ankle of your slide-side leg.
2. Keeping your weight primarily on the foot on the ground, slide the other foot backward, bending your knees and pausing when your back knee is just above the floor.
3. Push through your front leg to return to the starting position.
4. Complete the set on one side before repeating on the opposite leg.

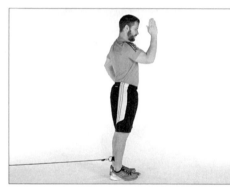 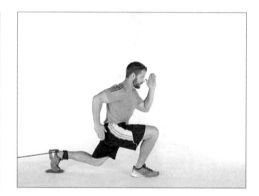

Split Squat Jump—Back Foot Elevated (Dumbbell)

STEPS

1. Place your back foot on a box or bench and step out into a lunge.
2. Lower your hips toward the floor by squatting back and down.
3. Without letting your back knee touch the ground, push off your front leg as powerfully as possible so that your front foot leaves the ground.
4. Complete the set on one side before repeating with the opposite leg forward.

COACHING KEY

Keep your back foot in contact with the bench by pushing down as you jump. Drive your elbows forward during the jump.

FEEL IT

Working your glutes, hamstrings, and quads.

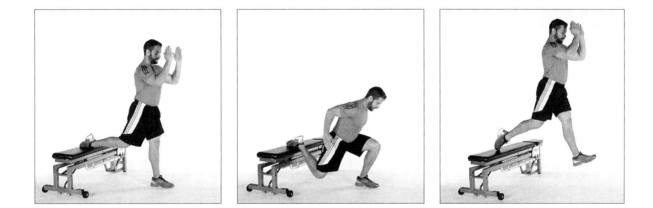

Split Squat—1 Arm (Dumbbell)

COACHING KEY

Keep most of your weight on your front foot with very little on your back foot.

FEEL IT

Working your glutes, hamstrings, and quads.

STEPS

1. Stand tall in a split stance with your feet shoulder-width apart and your weight primarily on the arch of your front foot. Hold a dumbbell down by your side with the same-side arm as your back leg.
2. Lower your hips toward the ground by bending your knees.
3. Without letting your back knee touch the ground, push through your front leg to return to the starting position.
4. Complete the set on one side before repeating with the opposite leg and arm.

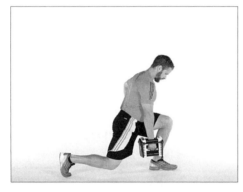 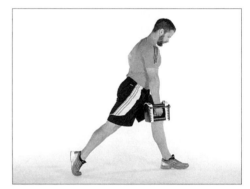

Split Squat—Back Foot Elevated (Dumbbell)

Maintain most of your weight on your front foot with very little on your back foot.

FEEL IT

Working your glutes, hamstrings, and quads.

STEPS

1. Holding dumbbells at arm's length at your sides, place your back foot on a box or bench and step out into a split stance.
2. Lower your hips toward the floor by squatting back and down.
3. Without letting your back knee touch the ground, push off your front leg to return to the starting position.
4. Complete the set on one side before repeating with the opposite leg.

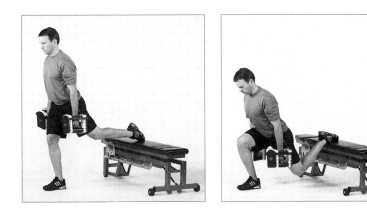

Squat—1 Leg Front-Loaded (Dumbbell)

1. Stand on one foot holding a pair of dumbbells on your shoulders with your elbows pointed out.
2. Initiating the move with your hips, squat back and down on one leg until your thighs are as close to parallel to the floor as possible.
3. Return to a standing position using only the leg you are balancing on.
4. Complete the set on one side before repeating with the opposite leg.

COACHING KEY

Keep your chest up and back flat, and do not let your knees collapse to the inside.

FEEL IT

Working your glutes, hamstrings, and quads.

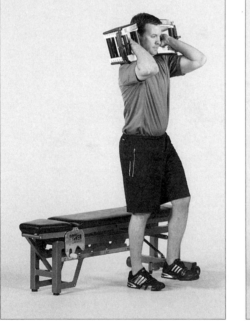
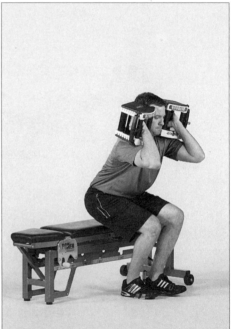

Leg Curl (Slide)

STEPS

1. Lie faceup on the floor with your arms at your sides, legs straight, and heels on a pair of slides (or on a towel on a slippery surface).
2. Lift your hips off the ground while keeping a straight line from your ankles to your shoulders.
3. Pull the slides toward your butt with your heels while keeping your hips tall.
4. Return to the starting position by slowly extending your legs and pushing the slides away from you.
5. Continue for the remainder of the set.

COACHING KEY

Initiate the movement by firing your glutes, keeping them contracted throughout the movement. Do not let your hips drop to the ground as you pull your heels toward your butt.

FEEL IT

Working your glutes, hamstrings, and lower back.

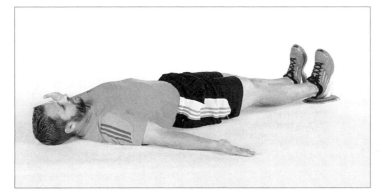

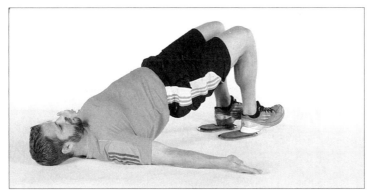

Leg Curl—1 Leg (Slide)

COACHING KEY

Initiate the movement by firing your glutes and keep them contracted throughout the movement. Keep your hips high off the ground as your heel moves toward your glutes.

FEEL IT

Working your glutes, hamstrings, and lower back.

STEPS

1. Lie faceup on the floor with your arms at your sides, one leg straight with the heel on a slide (or on a towel on a slippery surface), and your other hip and knee flexed to 90 degrees.
2. Lift your hips off the ground while keeping a straight line from your ankles to your shoulders as you pull the slide toward your glutes.
3. Return to the starting position by slowly extending your legs and pushing the slide away from you.
4. Complete the set on one leg before repeating on the other.

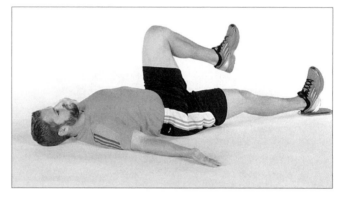

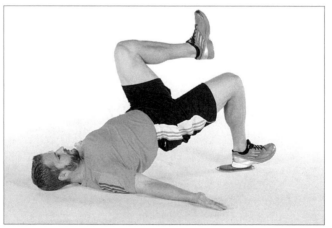

Leg Curl—1 Leg (Stability Ball)

STEPS

1. Lie faceup on the floor with your legs straight and your heels on top of a stability ball about shoulder-width apart.
2. Lift your hips until your body is in a straight line from your ankles to your shoulders.
3. Bend one hip to 90 degrees, lifting that leg off the ball.
4. Keeping your hips tall and your toes pulled toward your shin, pull the ball toward your butt with your heel.
5. Slowly extend your leg to push the ball away from you.
6. Complete the set on one side before repeating on the other side.

COACHING KEY

Keep your toes pulled toward your shin and do not let your hips drop as you pull your heel toward your butt.

FEEL IT

Working your glutes, hamstrings, and lower back.

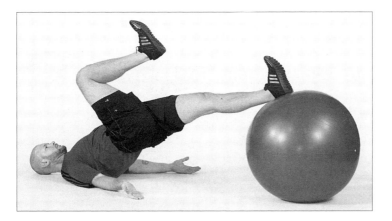

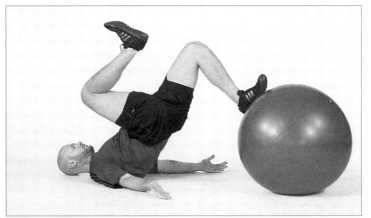

Leg Curl—Eccentric (Slide)

STEPS

1. Lie faceup on the floor with your arms at your sides, knees bent, and heels on a pair of slides (or on a towel on a slippery surface).
2. Pull your heels to your butt.
3. Contract your glutes to raise your hips, creating a straight line from your shoulders to your knees.
4. Straighten your legs in front of you in a slow, controlled motion.
5. Return to the starting position and repeat the movement.
6. Continue for the remainder of the set.

COACHING KEY
Initiate the movement by contracting your glutes.

FEEL IT
Working your glutes, hamstrings, and lower back.

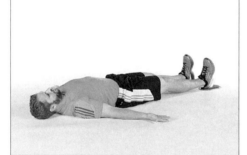
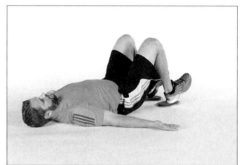
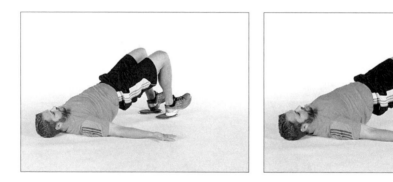

Romanian Deadlift [RDL] (Barbell)

STEPS

1. Stand holding a barbell with your hands just wider than shoulder-width.
2. Maintaining a flat back, hinge forward at the waist and lower the barbell, keeping it close to your shins.
3. Return to the standing position by contracting your hamstrings and glutes.
4. Continue for the full set.

COACHING KEY
Keep the bar close to your body throughout the movement.

FEEL IT
Working your glutes, hamstrings, and lower back.

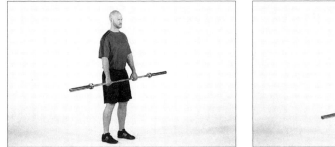
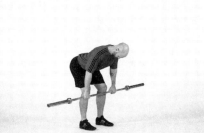

Romanian Deadlift [RDL] (Dumbbell)

STEPS

1. Stand with your knees slightly bent, holding a pair of dumbbells with an overhand grip (palms facing toward you).
2. Hinge forward at the waist, lowering the dumbbells toward your shins.
3. Contract your glutes and hamstrings to return to a standing position.
4. Continue for the full set.

COACHING KEY
Keep the dumbbells close to your legs, and keep your shoulder blades back and down throughout the movement.

FEEL IT
Working your glutes, hamstrings, and back.

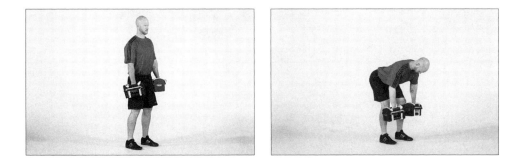

Romanian Deadlift [RDL] (Horizontal Band, Barbell)

COACHING KEY
Keep the bar close to your body throughout the movement.

FEEL IT
Working your glutes, hamstrings and lower back.

STEPS

1. Stand holding a barbell with your hands just wider than shoulder-width and a jump band around your waist with tension pulling behind you.
2. Maintaining a flat back, hinge forward at the waist and lower the barbell, keeping it close to your shins.
3. Return to the standing position by contracting your hamstring and glutes and pulling your hips forward against the tension of the band.
4. Continue for the full set.

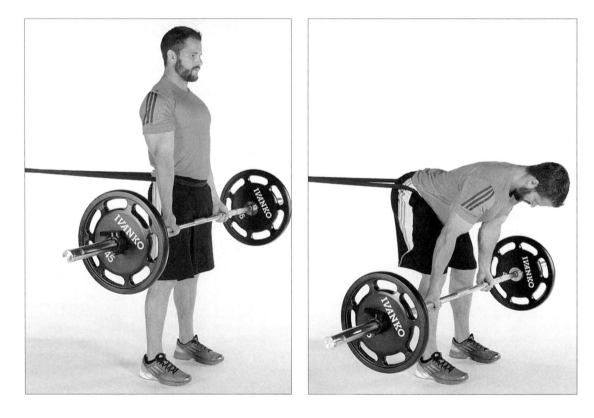

Romanian Deadlift [RDL] (Vertical Band, Barbell)

STEPS

1. Stand holding a barbell with your hands just wider than shoulder-width, standing on a jump band that is wrapped around both sides of the barbell.
2. Maintaining a flat back, hinge forward at the waist and lower the barbell, keeping it close to your shins.
3. Return to the standing position by contracting your hamstrings and glutes.
4. Continue for the full set.

COACHING KEY

Keep the bar close to your body throughout the movement.

FEEL IT

Working your glutes, hamstrings, and lower back.

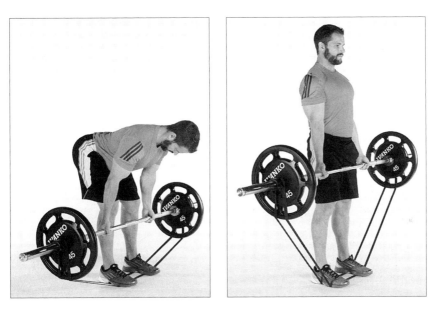

Romanian Deadlift [RDL]—1 Arm, 1 Leg (Dumbbell—Contralateral)

COACHING KEY

Move your torso and leg as one unit while keeping the weight close to your body throughout the movement.

FEEL IT

Working your glutes, hamstrings, and back.

STEPS

1. Stand on one foot with your knee slightly bent, holding a dumbbell in the opposite hand with an overhand grip (palm facing toward you).
2. Hinge forward at the waist, lowering the dumbbell as your non-supporting leg lifts behind you.
3. Contract your glutes and hamstrings to return to a standing position.
4. Complete the set on one side before repeating with the opposite leg and arm.

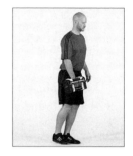

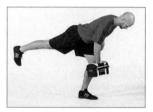

Romanian Deadlift [RDL]—2 Arm, 1 Leg (Dumbbell)

COACHING KEY

Move your torso and leg as one unit while keeping the weights close to your body throughout the movement.

FEEL IT

Working your glutes, hamstrings, and back.

STEPS

1. Stand on one foot with your knee slightly bent, holding dumbbells in each hand.
2. Hinge forward at the waist, lowering the weights as your non-supporting leg lifts behind you.
3. Contract your glutes and hamstrings to return to a standing position.
4. Complete the set on one side before repeating with the opposite leg.

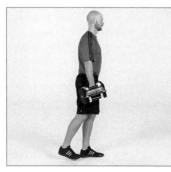

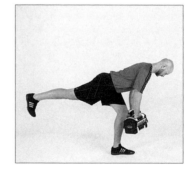

150-Yard Shuttle

STEPS

1. Stand in a split stance with your feet hip-width apart so one foot is in front of the other.
2. Sprint forward for 25 yards, turn around, and sprint back 25 yards.
3. Immediately turn around and repeat the sprint for 2 more laps, a total of 150 yards.
4. Rest for the designated amount of time and repeat.

300-Yard Shuttle

STEPS

1. Stand in a split stance with your feet hip-width apart so one foot is in front of the other.
2. Sprint forward for 25 yards, turn around, and sprint back 25 yards.
3. Immediately turn around and repeat the sprint for 5 more laps, a total of 300 yards.
4. Rest for the designated amount of time and repeat.

COACHING TIP
As you push off with one leg, drive the same-side arm forward and the opposite elbow back to help extend your hips and create a faster turnover.

FEEL IT
Working your entire body.

COACHING TIP
As you push off with one leg, drive the same-side arm forward and the opposite elbow back to help extend your hips and create a faster turnover.

FEEL IT
Working your entire body.

Ladder Shuttle Drill (5-10-15)

1. Stand in a split stance with your feet hip-width apart so one foot is in front of the other.
2. Sprint forward for 5 yards, turn around, and sprint back 5 yards.
3. Immediately turn around again, sprint for 10 yards, turn around, and sprint 10 yards back.
4. Immediately turn around again, sprint for 15 yards, turn around, and sprint 15 yards back.
5. Rest for the designated amount of time and repeat.

Ladder Shuttle Drill (5-10-15-20-25)

STEPS

1. Stand in a split stance with your feet hip-width apart so one foot is in front of the other.
2. Sprint forward for 5 yards, turn around, and sprint back 5 yards.
3. Immediately turn around again, sprint for 10 yards, turn around, and sprint 10 yards back.
4. Repeat this sprinting pattern for 15, 20, and then 25 yards.
5. Rest for the designated amount of time and repeat.

Sprint

1. Stand in a split stance with your feet hip-width apart so one foot is in front of the other.
2. Without stepping backward, drive through your hips and accelerate forward, maintaining a forward lean and good posture.
3. Continue to accelerate forward for the prescribed distance.
4. Rest for the designated amount of time and repeat.
5. Continue for the full set.

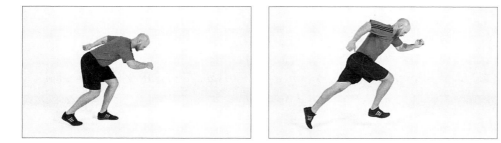

COACHING TIP
As you push off with one leg, drive the same-side arm forward and the opposite elbow back to help extend your hips and create a faster turnover.

FEEL IT
Working your entire body.

Your Choice (ESD)

STEPS

1. Pick any type of conditioning activity—running, swimming, the elliptical, or biking, for example.
2. Perform the activity for the prescribed amount of time at the designated effort.

COACHING KEY
Maintain proper technique as you become fatigued.

FEEL IT
Working your entire body.

90-90 Stretch with Arm Sweep

STEPS

1. Lie faceup with one knee bent at 90 degrees and the other leg crossed over top.
2. Roll onto the side of your bottom leg.
3. Keeping your bottom arm pinned to the ground, rotate your chest and top arm away, trying to place your back on the ground.
4. Extend the same arm and sweep it along the ground toward your head until it is straight overhead.
5. Sweep your arm down toward your butt.
6. Return to the starting position by reversing the movement.
7. Continue for the remainder of the set before repeating with the opposite side.

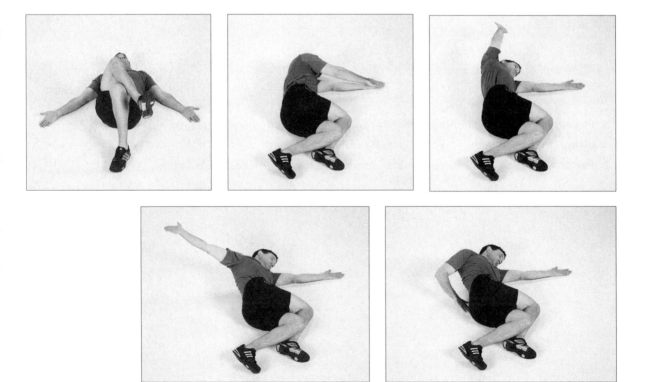

Abductor Stretch (Rope)

1. Lie on your back with a rope around one foot, wrapped around the outside of your ankle. Hold the ends of the rope in your opposite hand with your free hand out to the side.
2. Lift your leg across your body as far as possible. Then give gentle assistance with the rope until you feel a stretch. Hold for 2 seconds.
3. Relax and return to the starting position.
4. Complete the set on one side before repeating with the opposite leg.

COACHING KEY

Keep your non-roped leg on the ground by pushing your heel away from your head, contracting your glute, and pointing your toes toward the sky.

FEEL IT

Stretching the outside thigh of the roped leg.

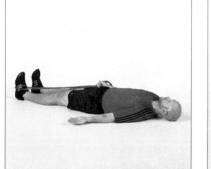
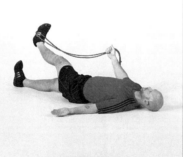
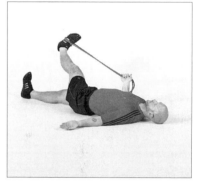

Adductor Stretch—Half Kneeling

1. Start in a half-kneeling position with your knee on a soft pad or mat. Rotate your knee-down leg in toward your body so your foot is outside the opposite hip.
2. With a slight forward lean of the torso, tighten your core and contract the glute of the knee-down leg.
3. Maintaining this position, gently shift your entire body slightly forward. Hold for 1 to 2 seconds.
4. Relax and return to the starting position.
5. Complete the set on one side before repeating on the opposite side.

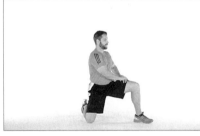 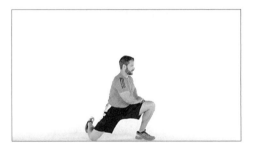

Bent-Knee Hamstring Stretch

STEPS

1. Lie on your back with both legs straight out on the ground. Pull one knee toward your chest, grasping behind the knee with both hands.
2. Straighten your bent leg toward the sky. Hold the stretch for 2 seconds.
3. Relax and return to the starting position.
4. Complete the set on one side before repeating with the opposite leg.

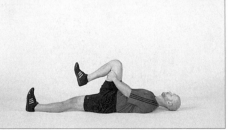 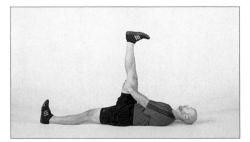

Foam Roll—Adductor

1. Lie facedown with a soft-tissue foam roll under the inside of one thigh and the other leg out to the side.
2. Roll along the inside of your thigh from your pelvis to the inside of your knee, spending more time rolling over any sore spots.
3. Complete the set on one side before repeating on the opposite leg.

COACHING KEY
Place as much weight on the foam roll as you can tolerate.

FEEL IT
Massaging your inner thigh.

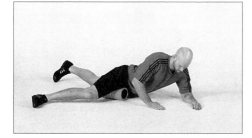
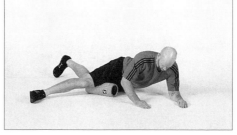

Foam Roll—Calf

1. Sit on the ground with your legs straight, one leg crossed over the other, and a soft-tissue foam roll under the calf of the bottom leg.
2. Lift your butt off the ground so that your weight is supported by your hands and the foam roll.
3. Keeping your hands still, move your body back and forth, rolling your lower leg over the foam roll, spending more time rolling over any sore spots.
4. Complete the set on one side before repeating on the opposite leg.

COACHING KEY
Place as much weight on the foam roll as you can tolerate.

FEEL IT
Massaging your calves.

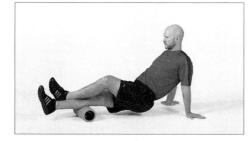
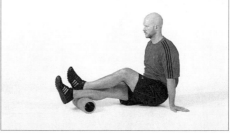

Foam Roll—Chest

1. Lie facedown with a foam roll under one side of your chest.
2. Roll along one side of your upper chest, spending more time rolling over any sore spots.
3. Complete the set on one side before repeating on the opposite side.

COACHING KEY
Place as much weight on the foam roll as you can tolerate.

FEEL IT
Massaging your chest.

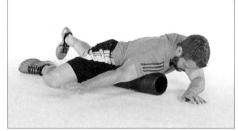
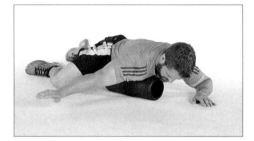

Foam Roll—Glutes

1. Sit on a foam roll with your weight shifted to one side and your hands and feet on the floor for support.
2. Roll from the top of the back of your thigh to your lower back, spending more time rolling over any sore spots.
3. Continue for the remainder of the set before repeating on the opposite side.

COACHING KEY
Place as much weight on the foam roll as you can tolerate.

FEEL IT
Massaging your glutes.

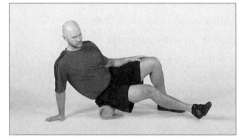
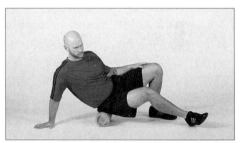

Foam Roll—Latissimus Dorsi

STEPS

1. Lie on your side with a foam roll under your armpit.
2. Roll along your side to your lower back and back up to your armpit, spending more time rolling over any sore spots.
3. Continue the set on one side before repeating on the opposite side.

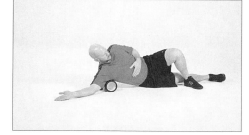

COACHING KEY
Place as much weight on the foam roll as you can tolerate.

FEEL IT
Massaging the side of your back.

Foam Roll—Low Back

STEPS

1. Lie on your side with a soft-tissue foam roll under one side of your lower back.
2. Roll from the middle of your back down to the base of your spine and back up, spending more time rolling over any sore spots.
3. Continue the set on one side before repeating on the opposite side.

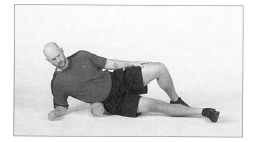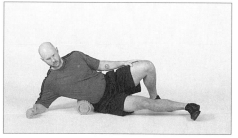

COACHING KEY
Place as much weight on the foam roll as you can tolerate.

FEEL IT
Massaging your lower back.

Foam Roll—Quadriceps

STEPS

1. Lie facedown on the ground, supporting your weight on your forearms with a foam roll under one thigh.
2. Roll along the quad from your hip to just above your knee, spending more time rolling over any sore spots.
3. For added benefit, roll the outside and inside as well as the front of the thigh.
4. Complete the set on one leg before repeating with the opposite leg.

COACHING KEY
Place as much weight on the foam roll as you can tolerate.

FEEL IT
Massaging the muscle of the front of the thigh and hip.

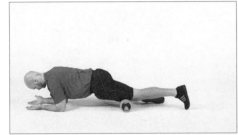
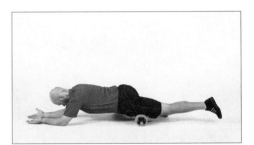

Foam Roll—Thoracic Spine

STEPS

1. Lie faceup on the ground with a foam roll under your upper back and your hands supporting your head.
2. Roll from the middle of your back up to the base of your neck and back down, spending more time rolling over any sore spots.
3. Continue for the full set.

COACHING KEY
Place as much weight on the foam roll as you can tolerate.

FEEL IT
Stretching your torso and middle and upper back.

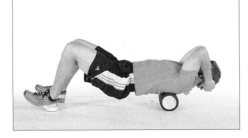
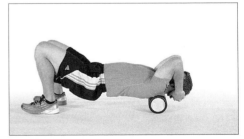

Foam Roll—Tibialis Anterior

STEPS

1. Start on your hands and knees with a foam roll under the front of your shins, just below your knees.
2. Keeping your hands still, pull your knees toward your hands and roll back and forth, spending more time rolling over any sore spots.
3. Continue for the remainder of the set.

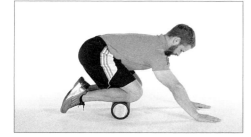
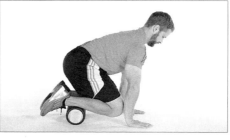

Foam Roll—Hamstrings

STEPS

1. Sit on the ground with your legs straight, one leg crossed over the other, and a foam roll under the thigh of the bottom leg.
2. Placing your hands on the ground behind you, lift your hips off the ground so that your weight is supported by your hands and the foam roll.
3. Keeping your hands still, move your body back and forth, rolling the length of your hamstrings from your knee to the top of your thigh, spending more time rolling over any sore spots.
4. Continue the set on one side before repeating on the opposite leg.

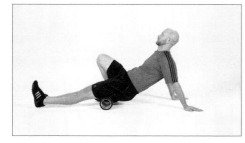
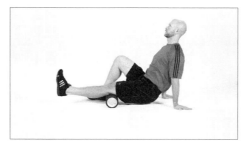

Foam Roll—IT Band

STEPS

1. Lie on your side supporting your weight on your forearm with a foam roll under your outer thigh.
2. Glide your body over the foam roll from your hip to just above the outside of your knee, spending more time rolling over any sore spots.
3. Continue for the remainder of the set before repeating with the opposite leg.

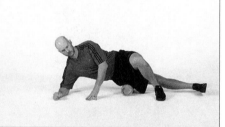
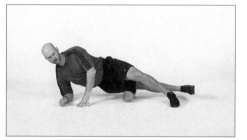

Inverted Hamstring with Rotation

STEPS

1. Stand on one leg and hold on to a support with the hand of the same side.
2. Hinge forward at your hip by dropping your chest and lifting your opposite leg to the ceiling to create a T with your body.
3. Rotate your hips and shoulders toward the ceiling until you feel a stretch on the inside of your hip. Hold it for 1 to 2 seconds.
4. Relax and rotate your hips back through the original T position until you feel a stretch on the outside of your hip.
5. Complete the set on one side before repeating on the other side.

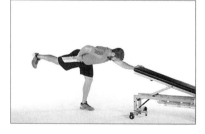
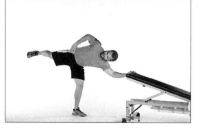
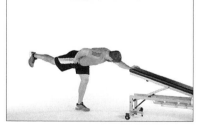

Massage Stick—Hamstrings

1. Sit holding a massage stick with a hand on either end.
2. Roll the stick back and forth quickly over all sides of the back of your thigh, from your glute down to behind your knee.
3. Complete the set on one leg before repeating on the opposite leg.

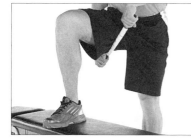 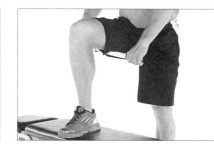

COACHING KEY

Use small oscillating motions and move up and down along the muscle. Spend more time on any sore spots that you find.

FEEL IT

Massaging the back of your thigh.

Massage Stick—Low Back

STEPS

1. Sit or stand holding a massage stick with a hand on either end.
2. Roll the stick back and forth quickly over the sides and middle of your lower back, from the bottom of your ribs to the top of your hips.
3. Continue for the full set.

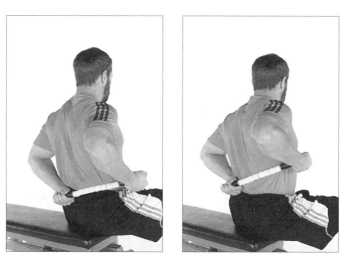

COACHING KEY

Use small oscillating motions and move up and down along the muscle. Spend more time on any sore spots that you find.

FEEL IT

Massaging your lower back.

Massage Stick—Neck

COACHING KEY
Use small oscillating motions and move up and down along the muscle. Spend more time on any sore spots that you find.

FEEL IT
Massaging your neck.

STEPS

1. Sit or stand holding a massage stick with a hand on either end.
2. Roll the stick back and forth quickly over the sides and back of your neck, from the top of your shoulders to the base of your skull.
3. Continue for the full set.

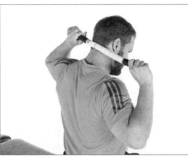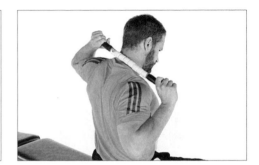

Massage Stick—Quadriceps

COACHING KEY
Use small oscillating motions and move up and down along the muscle. Spend more time on any sore spots that you find.

FEEL IT
Massaging the front of your thigh.

STEPS

1. Sit holding a massage stick with a hand on either end.
2. Roll the stick back and forth quickly over all sides of your quadriceps, from your hip down to your knee.
3. Complete the set on one leg before repeating on the opposite leg.

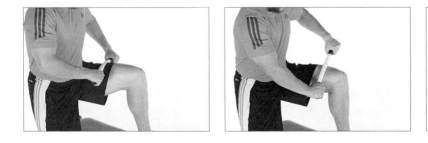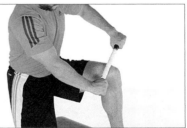

Massage Stick—TFL

STEPS

1. Sit holding a massage stick with a hand on either end.
2. Roll the stick back and forth quickly over the muscle on the outside of your upper thigh, just below the pelvis.
3. Complete the set on one leg before repeating on the opposite leg.

COACHING KEY

Use small oscillating motions and move up and down along the muscle. Spend more time on any sore spots that you find.

FEEL IT

Massaging the front of your hip.

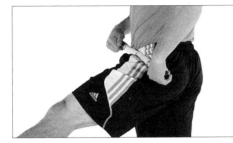 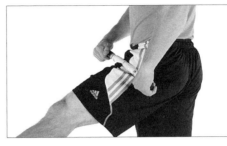

Quad/Hip Flexor Stretch—Half Kneeling

STEPS

1. Place one foot flat on the ground in front of you with your opposite knee on a soft pad or mat behind you. Grasp the thigh of your forward leg just above your knee.
2. Lean your torso slightly forward, tighten your stomach, and contract the glute of your back leg as you pull your arms away from your body.
3. Maintaining this position, hold for 2 seconds.
4. Relax and return to the starting position.
5. Complete the set on one side before repeating with the opposite foot forward.

COACHING KEY

Avoid arching your lower back.

FEEL IT

Stretching the front of the hip and the upper thigh of the back leg.

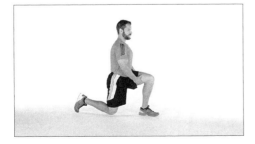 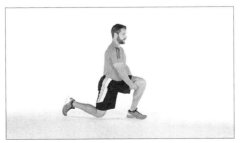

Quad/Hip Flexor Stretch—Half Kneeling with Lateral Flexion

STEPS

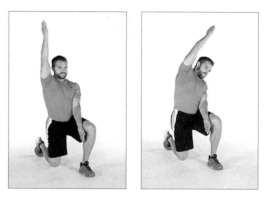

1. Place one foot flat on the ground and your opposite knee on a soft pad or mat with the hand of your kneeling side reaching over your head.
2. Lean slightly forward with your torso, tighten your stomach, and contract the glute of your back leg.
3. Maintaining this position, shift your entire body slightly forward.
4. Straighten your torso and return to the starting position.
5. Complete the set on one side before repeating with the other leg.

Quad/Hip Flexor Stretch—Sidelying

STEPS

1. Lie on your side with your knees pulled toward your chest, holding your top ankle with your top hand.
2. Pull the top leg back behind your body to feel a stretch in the front of your thigh and hip.
3. Hold for 2 seconds and return to starting position.
4. Complete set on one side before repeating on other.

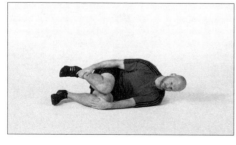
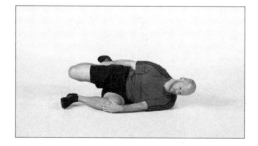

Reach, Roll, and Lift—Heel Sit (Foam Roll)

STEPS

1. Sit on your heels with your arms straight and your hands on a foam roll.
2. Roll the foam roll forward while keeping your hips back as your chest drops toward the floor. Hold for 2 seconds.
3. Relax and return to the starting position.
4. Continue for the remainder of the set.

COACHING KEY

Exhale as you roll the foam roll forward and try to rotate your palms to the ceiling.

FEEL IT

Stretching your upper back and shoulders.

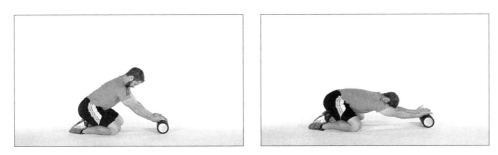

Sidelying Shoulder Stretch

STEPS

1. Lie on your side with your bottom arm perpendicular to your torso and your elbow bent 90 degrees.
2. Rotate your hand straight up and then toward the ground as far as possible while leaving your upper arm on the ground. Using your other hand to assist, gently press your hand farther and hold for 2 seconds.
3. Relax and return to the starting position.
4. Complete the set with one arm before repeating with the other arm.

COACHING KEY

Actively try to reach your palm to the ground throughout the stretch.

FEEL IT

Stretching your back and the shoulder closest to the ground.

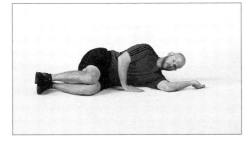
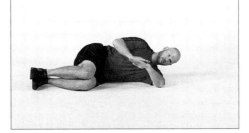

Sliding Overhead Press

1. Lie faceup on the ground with your hips and knees bent. Place your arms out to your sides with your elbows bent to 90 degrees, palms facing up, and hands pointed above your head.
2. Slide your arms overhead, keeping your hands on the ground.
3. Return to the starting position.
4. Continue for the remainder of the set.

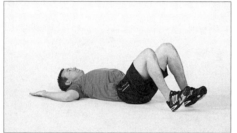
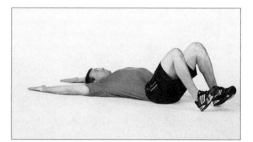

Supine Hip Rotator Stretch

STEPS

1. Lie faceup on the ground with your knees bent, arms extended out to the sides, feet wider than shoulder-width apart, and toes in the air and pointed up.
2. Rotate your hips inward by moving your legs toward each other while keeping your heels stationary. Hold for 2 seconds.
3. Relax and return to the starting position.
4. Continue for the remainder of the set.

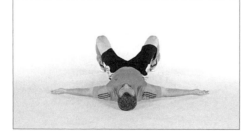
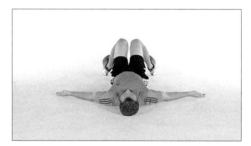

Trigger Point—Arch/Plantar Fascia

STEPS

1. Stand with your shoes off and one foot on a trigger ball (tennis ball, for example).
2. Roll the arch of your foot back and forth over the ball, holding on any sore spots you find.
3. Continue for the remainder of the set before repeating on the opposite foot.

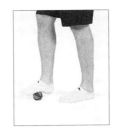

COACHING KEY
Maintain pressure on the ball throughout the set.

FEEL IT
Releasing tension in the arches of your feet.

Trigger Point—Glutes

STEPS

1. Sit with a trigger ball (tennis ball, for example) under the outside of one of your glutes with both knees slightly bent.
2. Adjust the position of the ball until you find a sore spot.
3. Holding pressure on this spot, slowly bend your hip up and down to release the tension.
4. Readjust your position on the ball and repeat the movement on any other sore spots you find.
5. Continue for the remainder of the set before repeating on the opposite leg.

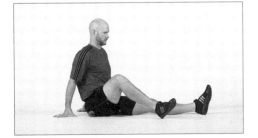 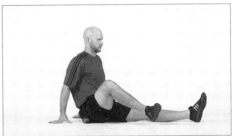

COACHING KEY
Adjust the pressure as tolerated by placing more weight through your arms and opposite leg. Maintain pressure on the ball throughout the set.

FEEL IT
Releasing tension in your hips.

Trigger Point—Neck

1. Lie on your back with your hips and knees bent with a double trigger ball (two tennis balls taped together, for example) just below the base of your head.
2. Adjust your position on the ball until you find a sore spot.
3. Hold on the spot and slowly nod your head up and down.
4. Continue for the remainder of the set.

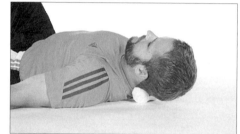
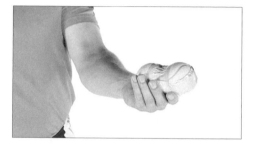

Trigger Point—TFL

STEPS

1. Lie facedown on the ground supported on your forearms with a trigger ball (tennis ball, for example) under one hip.
2. Roll along the front of the hip and slightly outside the upper thigh below the pelvis until you find a sore spot.
3. Hold on this spot for the prescribed amount of time and repeat on any other sore spots.
4. Repeat with the opposite leg.

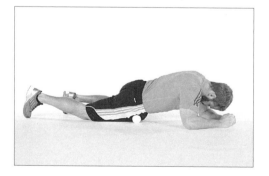

Trigger Point—Thoracic Spine

1. Lie on your back with a double trigger ball (two tennis balls taped together, for example) under your spine, just above your lower back. Place your hands behind your head.
2. Perform 3 crunches.
3. Raise your arms straight up over your chest, and then reach one arm overhead in an arc.
4. Return to the starting position and repeat with the other arm.
5. Continue alternating for 3 repetitions with each arm.
6. Move the double trigger ball up your spine 1 to 2 inches and repeat the crunches and arm reaches.
7. Continue moving the double trigger ball up your spine until it is just above your shoulder blades and below the base of your neck.

COACHING KEY

Take your time with each repetition, exhaling as you reach overhead.

FEEL IT

Releasing tension in your middle to upper back.

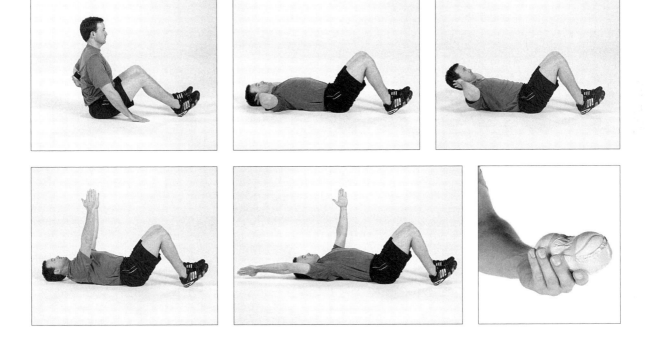

Trigger Point—VMO

FEEL IT

Releasing tension in your quadriceps.

STEPS

1. Lie facedown with a trigger ball (tennis ball, for example) under your VMO (the lower front of your inner thigh just above the knee).
2. Adjust your position on the ball until you find a sore point.
3. Holding pressure on this spot, slowly bend and extend your knee for the prescribed number of repetitions.
4. Readjust your position on the ball and repeat the movement on any other sore spots you find.

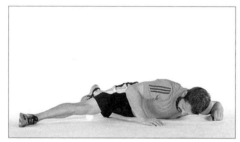 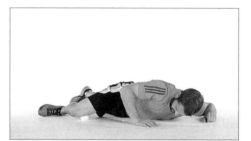

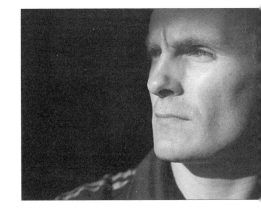

Afterword

IT IS INSPIRING WHEN HIGH PERFORMERS TURN EVERY ETHICAL STONE OVER TO learn and take their performances to a higher level. We are honored to be a small empowering part of your journey. We deeply respect your embodiment of the high-performance life, which many say is full of great sacrifice. What they don't understand is that when you are living your defined purpose, your IT, side by side with like-minded others you love and respect, it is far from a sacrifice. Indeed, it's the bull's-eye of a fulfilling life.

At EXOS, we feel a tremendous responsibility to help you achieve your IT. We continue to move forward every day with great unity and relentless determination, using our ingenuity to address every situation our athletes face with the utmost integrity and humility.

Please visit us at AthletesPerformance.com, where you can follow our latest developments. If you are the best at what you do, or well on your way to becoming it, plan on visiting one of our world-class facilities, where we'll work side by side to take your performance to the next level. If you are one of our

293

peers, we would be honored to share with you firsthand via one of our educational courses at one of our facilities around the world. There the best of the best in all related fields covered in this book give us a 95 percent excellence rating and are valued members of our EXOS community.

CorePerformance.com also is an excellent resource to find the latest research and insight related to Mindset, Nutrition, Movement, and Recovery, with thousands of supporting articles. It is also an excellent source to view every movement within this book and 1,800 additional exercise videos and descriptions. Our social media is very active and is a great resource to bring greater clarity to the contents of this book and the high-performance life. CorePerformance.com contains the majority of items needed to perform the exercises in this book, but you also can use Amazon.com, leading sport retailers, or whatever is available within your gym to find the tools to create your success. There are no excuses, just results.

We deeply appreciate our elite performers in the military who truly sacrifice for our country and our way of life. These inspiring people define the high-performance life. Thanks to each and every one who protects our freedoms.

Sincerely,

Mark Verstegen

Acknowledgments

ATHLETES' PERFORMANCE, THE COMPANY, WAS FOUNDED IN 1999, AND THIS book is a direct reflection of the systems that my colleagues and I have had the honor of developing and continuing to improve for elite tactical athletes as well as the top champions in sports. I'm fortunate to have been blessed with much of the same team throughout this ongoing journey.

Thank you to every one of our EXOS Teammates around the world, who have all contributed to the systems that empower our clients' success. Special thanks goes to our Performance Innovation Team leaders: Vice President Craig Friedman, Vice President Amanda Carlson, and Vice President Kevin Elsey, all of whom lead the collaboration with our Teammates across Mindset, Nutrition, Movement, and Recovery. A very special thank-you also goes to Anna Hartman, Dr. Roy Sugarman, Joe Gomes, Nick Winkelman, Darcy Norman, and Brett Bartholomew.

This book would not exist at all were it not for Avery editor Megan Newman, who brought us back for a second book and trusted us to deliver a title that took our successful Core Performance franchise up a notch.

David Black is the best literary agent in the business, an elite performer by any definition. Ditto for my tag team partner, Pete Williams, whom I met when Athletes' Performance was just blueprints and an idea. David and Pete were among the first to embrace the Athletes' Performance vision, and I'm forever grateful for their guidance and support.

Finally there's Amy Verstegen and our families, who have inspired me to levels of performance I never thought possible.

Bibliography

THE ATHLETES' PERFORMANCE TRAINING SYSTEM IS SUPPORTED BY THOUSANDS of research papers across the cognitive, physiologic, biochemical, biomechanical, and motor behavior sciences. It is outside the scope of this book to provide an exhaustive list of all this research. Below is a list of books and authors that have greatly influenced the AP Training System over the years.

- *Active Isolated Stretching*, Aaron Mattes
- *Advances in Functional Training*, Michael Boyle
- *Anatomy Trains*, Thomas Myers
- *Athletic Body in Balance*, Gray Cook
- *Attention and Motor Skill Learning*, Gabriele Wulf
- *Children & Sports Training*, Józef Drabik
- *Designing Strength Training Programs and Facilities*, Michael Boyle
- *Diagnosis and Treatment of Movement Impairment Syndromes*, Shirley Sahrmann

- *High-Performance Sports Conditioning*, Bill Foran (editor)
- *High-Powered Plyometrics*, James Radcliffe and Robert Farentinos
- *Jumping into Plyometrics*, Donald Chu
- *Lore of Running* (fourth edition), Timothy Noakes
- *Low Back Disorders* (second edition), Stuart McGill
- *Mind Gym*, Gary Mack with David Casstevens
- *Movement: Functional Movement Systems*, Gray Cook, Lee Burton, Kyle Kiesel, Greg Rose, and Milo Bryant
- *Movement System Impairment Syndromes of the Extremities, Cervical and Thoracic Spine*, Shirley Sahrmann
- *Nancy Clark's Sports Nutrition Guidebook* (fifth edition), Nancy Clark
- *Periodization: Theory and Methodology of Training* (fifth edition), Tudor Bompa and Gregory Haff
- *Principles and Practice of Resistance Training*, Michael Stone, Meg Stone, and William Sands
- *Running: Biomechanics and Exercise Physiology Applied in Practice*, Frans Bosch and Ronald Klomp
- *Starting Strength* (third edition), Mark Rippetoe
- *Strength and Conditioning: Biological Principles and Practical Applications*, Marco Cardinale, Robert Newton, and Kazunori Nosaka (editors)
- *Stretch to Win*, Ann Frederick and Chris Frederick
- *Take a Nap! Change Your Life*, Sara Mednick and Mark Ehrman
- *Ultimate Back Fitness and Performance* (fourth edition), Stuart McGill

For a complete list of all exercises included in *Every Day Is Game Day,* please consult
pages 139–141.

Active Isolated Stretching (AIS), 29,
133–34
dynamic, 133
for flexibility and mobility, 69–70, 133
static, 29, 69, 134–35
stretch-and-hold routines, 69–70
stretch-shortening cycle (SSC), 71
supplements. See nutritional
complements

T

targeted breathing, 24
template explanations
ESD (Energy Systems Development)
sessions, 91–92
Movement Skills sessions, 101–2
Power sessions, 98–101
templates
Movement Skills sessions, 110
Power sessions, 105–9
Regeneration sessions, 111
tempo
in breathing, 126–27, 128
in movement patterns, 88
thoracic spine function, 68
torso (core) stability, 67–68
transverse plane, 66
travel, nutritional strategies for, 51–52
trigger point exercises, 26, 76, 131–32
triple-threat position, 80

U

upper cross syndrome, 65

V

visualization of IT benefits, 14–15, 23, 25,
27, 28, 123
vitamin supplements, 24, 52–53

W

warm-ups
as investment, 7
Movement Prep, 69–71
Pillar Prep, 64–69
stretch-and-hold routines, 69–70
workouts
Complementary sessions, 96–97,
103
components, 98
Energy Systems Development (ESD)
sessions, 94–95, 102–3
equipment, 96
in morning hours, 24
Movement Skills sessions, 92, 101–2
Movement Skills session template,
110
postworkout fueling, 28, 43, 49–50
Power sessions and microcycles,
93–101
Power session templates, 105–9
preworkout fueling, 28, 48
Regeneration sessions, 103
Regeneration session template, 111

Z

zone performance, 128

MARK VERSTEGEN pioneered the concept of integrated performance training and over the last fifteen years has brought that system to the world's top
athletes, teams, and sports organizations; the United States military; and leading companies, such as Intel, Walgreens, LinkedIn, and Sheraton Hotels and
Resorts. As president of EXOS, formerly Athletes' Performance and Core Performance, he leads more than five hundred employees at the company's training centers in Arizona, California, Florida, and Texas, as well as supplying
international support to top athletes and organizations. The athletes supported
by EXOS have received nearly every accolade in sports, and the world's
most forward-thinking companies rely on EXOS to motivate, educate, and engage their employees. Verstegen is the author of five books, including *Core
Performance*, which popularized integrated performance training and has sold
more than two hundred thousand copies. His widely acclaimed Core Performance system is also available online through interactive programs and other
world-class performance lifestyle content at CorePerformance.com. Verstegen

and EXOS consult for high-performance companies including Adidas, EAS, SKLZ, Keiser, and Axon Sports, helping them with product and program inspiration, development, and testing, as well as consumer marketing. EXOS has also partnered with the Mayo Clinic to advance proactive health and human performance. Verstegen serves as the director of performance for the NFL Players Association, where he focuses on player safety and welfare. He's regularly interviewed for training insight for publications and is a sought-after industry speaker who regularly presents at the leading conferences in the field. The Washington native lives in Phoenix, Arizona.

PETE WILLIAMS has worked with Mark Verstegen for more than a decade, coauthoring Verstegen's groundbreaking book *Core Performance* and four subsequent titles, and contributing regularly to CorePerformance.com. A NASM-certified personal trainer and a former *USA Today* sportswriter, Williams has authored and coauthored a number of other books, including *Obstacle Fit*, a training program focused on preparing for obstacle course races. The Virginia native and avid endurance athlete lives in Central Florida. His website is www.petewilliams.net.

ALSO AVAILABLE BY MARK VERSTEGEN

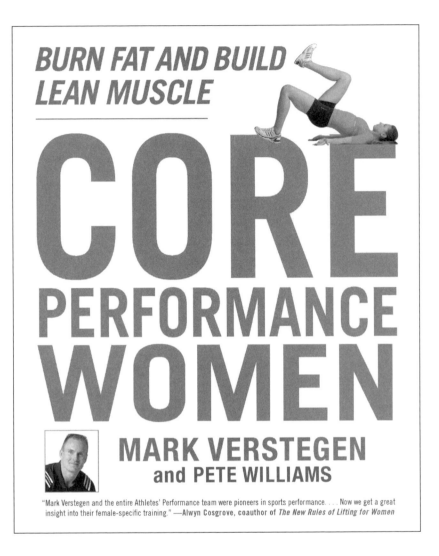

BURN FAT AND BUILD LEAN MUSCLE

CORE
PERFORMANCE WOMEN

MARK VERSTEGEN
and PETE WILLIAMS

"Mark Verstegen and the entire Athletes' Performance team were pioneers in sports performance. . . . Now we get a great insight into their female-specific training." —Alwyn Cosgrove, coauthor of *The New Rules of Lifting for Women*

Get fit with Verstegen's high-performance method targeted specifically for women.

AVERY